P9-DNU-161

CURVY YOGA

CURVY YOGA

Love Yourself
& Your Body
a Little More
Each Day

Anna Guest-Jelley

STERLING
New York

STERLING
New York

An Imprint of Sterling Publishing Co., Inc.
1166 Avenue of the Americas
New York, NY 10036

Sterling and the distinctive Sterling logo are
registered trademarks of Sterling Publishing Co., Inc.

© 2017 by Anna Guest-Jelley

All rights reserved. No part of this publication may be reproduced,
stored in a retrieval system, or transmitted in any form or by any means
(including electronic, mechanical, photocopying, recording, or otherwise)
without prior written permission from the publisher.

ISBN 978-1-4549-2066-3

Library of Congress Cataloging-in-Publication Data
Names: Guest-Jelley, Anna, author.
Title: Curvy yoga / Anna Guest-Jelley.
Description: New York, New York : Sterling Publishing, [2017]
Identifiers: LCCN 2016034279 | ISBN 9781454920663 (paperback)
Subjects: LCSH: Yoga--Psychological aspects. | Exercise--Popular works. |
    BISAC: HEALTH & FITNESS / Yoga. | HEALTH & FITNESS / Exercise.
Classification: LCC RA781.67 .G84 2017 | DDC 613.7/046--dc23
LC record available at https://lccn.loc.gov/2016034279

Distributed in Canada by Sterling Publishing Co., Inc.
c/o Canadian Manda Group, 664 Annette Street
Toronto, Ontario, Canada M6S 2C8
Distributed in the United Kingdom by GMC Distribution Services
Castle Place, 166 High Street, Lewes, East Sussex, England BN7 1XU
Distributed in Australia by NewSouth Books
45 Beach Street, Coogee, NSW 2034, Australia

For information about custom editions, special sales, and
premium and corporate purchases, please contact Sterling Special Sales
at 800-805-5489 or specialsales@sterlingpublishing.com.

Manufactured in China

2 4 6 8 10 9 7 5 3 1

www.sterlingpublishing.com

Design by Christine Heun
Photographs courtesy of Emily Gnetz

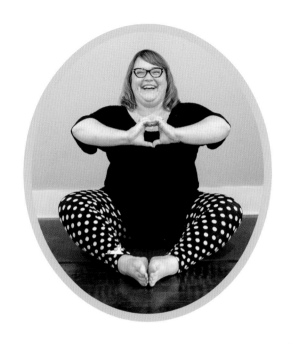

This book is for anyone who ever had
a negative thought about his or her body
and wondered, even just for a second,
if there could be another way.

CONTENTS

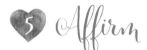
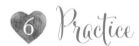

Preface

After practicing body acceptance for a few years, I almost threw it all out the window in the blink of an eye—for the promise of easy and virtually guaranteed weight loss.

All I had to do was inject myself with some urine by-product and only consume five hundred calories each day.

I know. I'd lived so long by the dieter's motto (if it sounds too good to be true . . . better try it) that even I'm not sure how I passed up that sweet deal.

One of the things that happens when you're curvy (regardless of your size in most cases) is that going to the doctor is a total roll of the dice. In my own experience, I have often been shamed—both subtly and not so subtly.

What I haven't often been, though, is heard. But then I met a doctor who befriended me. Our bodies didn't look too dissimilar from each other, so I felt a kinship with her. She shared her story of being on many different diets over the years, which I totally related to as I shared some stories of my own.

At this point, the conversation had been so easy and fun that I thought we were possibly destined to be besties. So when she started to tell me about this natural diet she'd been on that had caused her to lose more weight than she ever had before, how it's the only thing she'd ever researched that *actually* works, how it's natural, you better believe my ears perked right up.

And the good news? All I had to do was give myself the aforementioned injections of a hormone contained in pregnant women's urine and limit myself to five hundred calories a day. "It's totally easy," she said, "you won't even be hungry!"

She had me hook, line, and sinker. Of course I wouldn't go on a fad diet. How passé! But something 'natural'? That wasn't FDA approved only because it would have ruined the diet industry (gotta love a diet conspiracy theory, right)? That a doctor I knew and liked and seemed a lot like me recommended? Sounds awesome!

Okay, I realize it may sound completely ridiculous. It does to me now. But after decades of hearing messages about how unsafe and terrible my body was, I believed it. And why wouldn't I? Everyone from doctors to family to friends to media to pretty much everyone else agreed.

So injecting a little urine by-product and starving myself? Sounded like a pretty smart move to me if I could finally, finally lose weight and have the dream life I'd always imagined would magically accrue to me the moment I got thin.

When I met this doctor and considered the diet, my work on body acceptance had begun but clearly still had a long way to go. Part of the difficulty in accepting your body shows itself when an opportunity comes out of nowhere that you just can't pass up. The more I thought about the diet, the harder and harder it became to ignore the old voice inside me. That voice telling me that despite many unsuccessful diets, this diet—this might-as-well-be-urine injection—yeah, this could be it.

I was hooked by the doctor's story because it was the same one I'd been telling myself, and that other people had been telling me, for decades. It's the story of a body only being acceptable if it looks and weighs a certain amount. Of weight loss at all costs, other health consequences be damned. (Because if a thin person said they were only eating five hundred calories a day, people would be extremely concerned. But fat people are often encouraged to do things like that, despite the obvious detriments.) Of never being good enough, regardless of anything I accomplished, if I couldn't lose weight. Of thinking to myself with each new diet, "This time will be different."

After considering the diet for a month or so—spending countless hours reading stories about it on the Internet, making an appointment to see the doc about it, cancelling the appointment then reconsidering, and seeing if I could just buy the injections online—I finally got off the fence and moved forward in the way I knew I had to, despite so much telling me I shouldn't and that I was an idiot to do so.

As you already know, I didn't do it. Not because I didn't want to (I did! Oh, how I did!), but because this time the words coming out of my mouth were different. This time, I said no. This time, I said I couldn't put my body through this. This time, I trusted my gut, which said that I hadn't done all that work on learning to love and trust myself and my body to be undone by some expensive pee injections.

And even though it took me well over a month to land there, I knew something fundamental had changed in me when I did. Because even a year before—not to mention three or five or ten or twenty—you better believe I would have been first in line to put those thousands on my credit card (because you *know* it wasn't cheap) and get started. I don't even have to wonder if that would have been true because I'd already done it for many other harebrained weight-loss plans in the past.

But this time, I checked in with my body repeatedly, doing the practice we'll discuss later in this book, and a different story took hold.

Oh, and remember that doc who almost convinced me to do this? At the end of her telling me about it, as a whispered aside, she mentioned that she'd gained all the weight back. But she assured me that was only temporary because she was going to start again soon—and that this time would be different.

What Came Before

The new story I began living started with a simple question: What if dieting, never saying a good thing about my body, always trying to change it, isn't the right approach at all? What if this isn't the way? It was a question that seemed innocuous enough on the surface—but only because I didn't realize how it would eventually crumble the entire foundation on which I'd built my relationship (or lack thereof) with my body.

Although body acceptance had been part of my life off and on for a few years at the point this new diet came my way, I hadn't yet really started living it (a small part of me kept secretly hoping that accepting my body would be the way that I'd finally lose all the weight for real).

But when I asked myself if there was another way to relate to my body, I began to question everything related to my relationship with my body. Mostly, I questioned what I wanted from losing weight. For so long it had been a given for me. "Lose weight = happiness" was all but tattooed on my face. But the longer I struggled, the more I started to wonder: Is that actually true? And also, what if I could just start being happy right now?

When my work with body acceptance first started, I'd been practicing yoga for almost a decade. Though I definitely didn't start it for any body acceptance reasons (I had chronic migraines at the time, and someone told me it might help), I began to realize how yoga had been laying a path for me all along. Not so much because achieving any certain pose was empowering but because yoga asked me to feel what was going on in my body, which, after a lifetime of letting diets dictate what I ate, how I moved my body, and even how I thought about myself, was all but impossible at first. But by the time I became interested in accepting my body, I was starting to catch the most fleeting glimpses of what a positive relationship with my body could be like. Because that, to me, is what body acceptance is—it's not giving up on your body or not taking care of it, as some people think and fear, but rather an ongoing and evolving conversation with your body. It's getting to know and respond to your body *more*, not less.

And though I would have never suspected it at the beginning, what I now see as the interconnected practices of yoga and body acceptance helped me begin to write a new story about my body and my life, one that shifted my focus from an adversarial relationship with my body to a friendly one, from only exercising or practicing yoga intermittently when I felt guilty about something I ate to making movement a sustainable practice, from having so many of my moments and memories laced with thoughts like "I hate myself," "I'd be better off dead," or horrible criticisms of each part of my body to rarely thinking *about* my body at all and instead being in a relationship *with* my body.

Through both body acceptance and yoga, I have found peace within myself in so many ways—and continue to do so. But there's nothing special about me that made this possible; what made it possible is following this simple practice and returning to it over and over again. You've got this, and this book is here to be the friend you call when you need a reminder.

Curvy Yoga Practice

I hate it when people say things like "Love your body!" or even "Every body can do yoga!" and then leave it at that. Encouragement isn't bad, but it's also not enough. I wrote this book because I want these practices of body acceptance and yoga to be regular parts of your life and not only exist in the realm of the abstract. My hope is that through the stories and examples you read, you find strategies and ideas to consider that you can apply to your actual life.

Each chapter of this book takes you through a different component of yoga, body acceptance, and how the two are woven together. This is not a step-by-step book because coming into a more positive relationship with your own body is not a step-by-step process in the linear sense. Instead, this book reflects the back-and-forth process and opens some doorways of possibility so you can consider which doors are best for you to walk through first.

Whether you are brand-new to the practice of yoga or an experienced practitioner, this book will help you find a useful lens for looking at your practice, support for the journey into awareness, and practical tools to make the poses work for *your* unique body. Despite the common idea that yoga practitioners are all about oneness, there are many different viewpoints about what yoga is, what it should be, and much more. In this book I don't unpack all of those details (I'd need another book!) or look in-depth at yoga history or philosophy. I focus on the connections between yoga and body acceptance and offer you some ways to see how they might work for your life.

The same is true whether this is the first day you've considered the idea of accepting your body or if you've been working with the process for a while. And as with yoga, I don't get into all the different ways people envision and live body acceptance. My focus here is on the connection with yoga and helping you find *your* way. Because, though they're often seen solely as the domain of people with societally preferred bodies, yoga and body acceptance are practices that are available to everyone. But since including yoga pose options for curvy bodies isn't yet the norm in most yoga classes, this book will give you those tools, too, so you know you have your own back in any yoga class or in your home practice.

This Book Is For You

If you're reading about this practice and thinking something like "Sure, that sounds good, but *I* can never accept *this* body," I hear you. I thought the same thing for most of my life. In fact, I wasn't even that generous; I would have found the whole idea so absurd as to be impossible. But somewhere deep down, I was desperate for another way.

Maybe you are, too?

If you are, or even if you think you might be a tiny bit one day, here's what I want you to know: You're not alone. While there will invariably be fits and starts (probably mostly fits at first) on your journey, it *is* possible to start living and enjoying your life right now in the body you have. You don't have to wait until you get that body you think you "should" have. Actually, I suspect you've already been waiting on that more than long enough, just like I had been, so it's more accurate to say you don't have to wait any longer.

Here's one thing I want you to consider: What do *I* want from losing weight (or however you may be wanting to change your body)? I'm serious.

Really think about it. You can even pause here, go write about it for a bit, and come back. I'll still be here.

What did you find? Here are some of the things I wanted when I really dug down beneath what I *thought* I wanted, like to wear a certain size, see the look of surprise on the face of someone who had shamed me when I finally showed up on their doorstep thin, or even to move my body with more ease: inner peace, relief, happiness, freedom. I think these are the things many of us want, and they're definitely what I want for you.

When I realized what I really wanted, I saw how I'd been looking in the wrong place for it all along. What I thought I wanted from a diet is what I got from the practices of body acceptance and yoga. On its own, yoga can be a path to better knowing and cultivating a relationship with yourself, and the same is true of body acceptance. So when you put them together, you have a potent combination for transforming your relationship with your body and yourself.

We're told there's some kind of magical formula inside weight loss, but ask anyone who has lost weight and still ends up hating their body or gains the weight back as the vast majority of people do, and they'll tell you—it's not true. The magic is in being at peace with yourself no matter your size. Because when you have that peace, you're free to take care of yourself however you need and then your weight just does what it does. With this approach, you're not treating yourself like your own medical patient or uncooperative student but as a human with needs you can learn how to meet. You and your body are knowable and wise, despite the many messages you may have received to the contrary.

Fortunately, more and more research is finally telling us the truth—that diets don't work and never have. The body has its own processes in place outside our ideas about what it should or shouldn't do. So when you go on a diet, your body actively works against you to retain the calories it's losing by increasing your appetite among other mechanisms. The good news is that studies show that healthy behaviors are what matter more to health than weight.[1] With the space to do what helps you feel your best without an obsessive focus on weight, it's surprising how much enjoyment you can find in finally getting to discover new things about yourself and what you need, like the movement you might like after all (swimming and hiking for me) and what you only did because you thought it was a good way to burn calories but you actually hate (treadmill for me). The same is true with food: I used to eat quite a bit of carrots and celery sticks because every diet for miles told me they were "good" snacks, but with the freedom to explore other foods, I realized that I don't actually like them at all. So I found new foods I do like!

This practice has helped me move from being the person who would rather die than be caught in a bathing suit to someone who swims laps several times per week at her local pool. From being someone who hid in the back of yoga rooms (when I actually worked up the courage to go) to teaching people all over the world. From being chronically unhappy and disembodied to enjoying the simple pleasures of fresh fruit, the wind on my face, and the way I fit in my favorite pants (which are definitely not the size I'd been planning on in my fantasy life).

I didn't change a thing *about* my body to do this. But I did change how I *relate* to my body thanks to this practice: presence, get curious, challenge, and affirm, both on and off the yoga mat.

And that has made all the difference.

There is nothing more radical than living in, embracing, and yes, even loving your body when the world tells you that's not okay. Nothing subverts a power structure like people rejecting it.

So let's go do some reimagining.

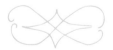

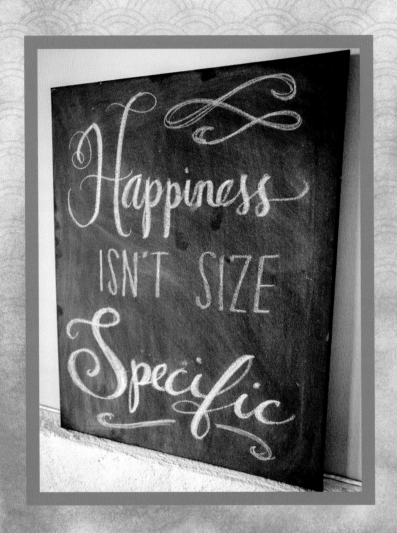

Twenty Years.
Sixty-Five Diets. No Results.

Or How We Got Here

Before I could write a new story about my own body, I first had to uncover my old story. One of my biggest continually unfolding discoveries was, and continues to be, how many of my stories reflect just how deeply and long I stewed in shame about my body.

The first time I vividly remember experiencing shame about my body (though I wouldn't have called it that at the time) was when I saw my middle school math teacher at a popular weight loss meeting.

That, in and of itself, is not too surprising—seeing a middle-aged woman at a weight loss meeting is pretty much par for the course. But the fact that I was still in middle school when it happened?

Yeaaaaaaah. That was hardly the norm. At least not at the time.

Here's how it went down: This was the early '90s, so my uniform was fluorescent bike shorts paired with an oversized fluorescent T-shirt (preferably with puffy paint). I also had my hair in a coordinating scrunchy, but you probably already guessed that.

The only meetings I was able to attend (since I needed someone to drive me and had, you know, to go to school) were also at the busiest times for the adult members: evenings or weekends. And since I had my aerobics class on weeknights (also populated with adults), I had to go on Saturday morning.

When I opened the door to the building on this particular Saturday, a tidal wave of women's voices washed over me. I always tried my best not to talk to anyone while I was there, but it seemed as if everyone else was chatting as much as possible, perhaps in hopes of burning a few extra calories before jumping on the scale. If you've never experienced this before, getting your turn for the weekly weigh-in is a little like the adult (or kid, in my case) version of going to the principal's office when you don't know why you've been called in. You're not yet sure if this is a "You're awesome and I just wanted to tell you" visit or an "I have something I need to talk to you about" visit.

As I crept closer to my turn on the scale, I felt alternately excited (how much have I lost?!) and anxious (how much have I lost?!). At twelve, this is a highly confusing experience. I didn't know how to name this simultaneous feeling of dread, anticipation, and wishing I could disappear through the floor regardless. All I knew is that if the scale showed a loss, I would make my mother happy, and we might go shopping afterward.

And if it didn't, the silence on the ride home would be deafening, even though it would also be occasionally peppered with overly enthusiastic questions about whether I needed some help tracking what I ate during the week.

By that point in my life, I'd already been in and out of dieting mode for several years, minimum. What had come before, unbranded calorie restriction, had always been supervised by my mom and my pediatrician, so this was my first time truly stepping into Diet World. (That has to be a place, right? After raking in an estimated $64 billion in 2014,[1] you'd think they could afford to build it.)

Finally, my moment of (hopeful) glory had arrived. I tiptoed into the cubicle, stepped delicately onto the scale, and held my breath (because what if breath caused me to gain 0.0001 pounds?!).

Not many good things happen to you when you're in middle school. You probably remember that, right? I was neither popular nor unpopular as a middle schooler (or, really, as a person at any point in my life). I mostly blended into the background, content to go to class and hang out with my small group of friends.

So when I heard the woman reading the scale declare that I'd lost a pound and a half (0.7 kg), it was with no small amount of glee that I grinned and looked up at my mom.

Vindication!

And this time, not only had I lost, but I'd reached one of this group's many celebrated milestones (because if they do one thing right, it's getting folks hooked on the intermittent rewards of weight loss): ten pounds (4.5 kg) down.

I was about to get a freakin' ribbon, y'all. No middle school field day competition required. (Thank goodness, since, as I'm sure you can already suspect, those competitions weren't exactly my forte.)

As I turned to leave the cubicle, still beaming, I paused mid-pivot, like one of those slow-mo scenes in the movies when you know everything is about to change. And probably not for the better.

Because at that moment I saw my math teacher. Not even a teacher from the past, but my current teacher. The one I'd have to see on Monday morning.

A pit dropped in my stomach, and I suddenly found myself dry-mouthed and spaced-out. I *had* to get out of there.

There was only one problem: my mom.

I couldn't get out of there without her, but I also couldn't possibly tell her what had happened. I mean, I already felt humiliated enough, always being the youngest person there by at least a decade, and usually more like two, three, or more. The thought of admitting to being "found out" was too much to bear.

So I decided then and there to do what I did best: blend in. I convinced my mom to take a seat with me near the back. Blessedly, since it was so jam-packed, people soon filled in around us, and we became nearly unnoticeable. I tracked my teacher out of the corner of my eye like a hawk and was relieved to see her find a seat in the front right of the room, far from our back left.

Or, at least it seemed far at the moment.

Before I knew it, we were through the meeting's lecture portion and on to the sharing time. In a flash, my mom elbowed me to jump in, encouraging me to share my victory with the woman leading the meeting. My attempts to brush off my mom, of course, caught the meeting leader's well-trained eye, and she asked me if I had something I'd like to share. I had one of those moments when a thousand options pass through your mind, none of them good. Should I act as if I didn't know whom she was talking to? Fake an illness? Kick the shin of the lady next to me to create a distraction?

As I felt my mom's elbow coming for me again, I squeaked out, "I lost ten pounds." I looked up at the leader helplessly, hoping against hope she'd see the desperation on my face and quickly move on to someone else, ready to celebrate their success or declare their recommitment.

Misinterpreting my facial expression as one that wanted public acknowledgment, the leader started the group in a round of ever-growing applause and whipped out my "ten pounds lost" ribbon faster than I could look away from my middle school teacher, who'd of course turned her head to me when I spoke.

It was, after all, still fairly rare to hear a young girl's voice in the room in those days.

As we made eye contact, I knew I'd never forget the look on her face: a mix of embarrassment for me and—yep, I saw it—jealousy. I mean, I'd lost ten pounds (4.5 kg).

Who wouldn't want that?

When I look back at that experience, I certainly don't see it as a moment of triumph. And despite feeling good about winning the approval of the adults around me, I wasn't even happy in that moment. I should have been: I'd achieved something I'd been working toward with a prize and accolades to boot (I'm sure I'll never receive that enthusiastic a round of applause again). Instead, I just felt really uncomfortable in my skin, as if I couldn't wait until all eyes and attention were off me. The feeling I had then of wanting to run away and hide wasn't a new one, though it was the first time I'd noticed it so strongly, and this was far from the last time I'd feel it.

This disappear-into-the-floor feeling is one that I now recognize as shame. Which, as Dr. Brené Brown,[2] a shame researcher, points out, isn't compatible with happiness. Why would I feel shame deep down in this moment? Because a feeling of my body never being good enough was always at the root of all of my weight loss endeavors. So even if I lost a little weight here or there, that feeling never went away. I lived in near constant fear of not having lost enough, gaining back what I had lost, or needing to lose more. Those three looped in my mind ceaselessly. So it's not too surprising how I felt during that weight loss meeting. Nor is it surprising that it took me decades to untangle my body from the web of shame it had gotten stuck in.

After all, the diet industry is predicated on one idea that persists against all logic and reason even though it is a multibillion-dollar industry whose products fail the vast majority of the time (95%)[3]: The problem isn't them—it's you. This is a system whose business plan is keeping all of us in shame as long as possible—hopefully our whole lives. And shame thrives in silence, which means we continue to blame ourselves for what in reality is a broken system that not only benefits from but actually requires our failure in order to ensure repeat customers. And why wouldn't we? Going on yet another diet, cooking up new ways to control our bodies, and putting ourselves down aren't signs of a different kind of failure in how we relate to ourselves; they're the natural response to a culture that tells us that we won't be acceptable unless we do.

We haven't failed. We've *been* failed.

And now we get to do something about it.

Where It All Began

I'd landed at that weight loss meeting in middle school because of a confluence of a few things: my pediatrician shaming my mother about my weight, my parents' own fear of fat (that, of course, grew out of their own upbringing), my growing body, and binge-eating. I'm not entirely sure when I started binge-eating, but I know it was in early elementary school if not before.

Even though my mother was hypervigilant about my weight, food (especially dessert) was plentiful in our house and somehow, shockingly, never hidden behind lock and key.

When you're an adult, binge-eating is relatively easy—you can drive/walk/take a bus somewhere, eat surreptitiously by yourself, and throw the wrapper away before you even get back home.

You have at least some access to the essential ingredients: time, money, and a getaway car.

As a kid, though, you have to be stealthy. So I got *really* good at knowing when I could sneak food, where I could hide it, and when I could eat it. When I say that I was *really* good, one thing you need to know is that my mom was a stay-at-home mom, and she was *involved*—usually way more than I might have liked.

Looking back, I'm not quite sure how I managed to sneak food, but I did. And I knew exactly what could slip away unnoticed (or at least unconfronted) and what couldn't. Half a sleeve of opened crackers? No: She'd remember there were more in there last time. But a whole sleeve?

Yes: She'd think she'd just forgotten how many sleeves were left. Cookies from the top of the tin? No: She'd wonder where they'd all gone. But a whole layer directly under the top layer? Yes, ma'am.

I became adept at jamming heaping spoonfuls of last night's leftovers into my mouth while she was in the bathroom—facing the fridge, of course, so I could pretend I was contemplating a snack and buy an extra second to swallow if she came back earlier than I was expecting.

I learned how to filch a piece of candy here or there, put it in my pocket, and deposit it under my bed throughout the day—until I had a nice li'l stash to enjoy by myself once I went to bed, the results of which I could dispose of discreetly the next day. I had to resort to this approach because as an even younger girl I'd tossed the trash behind the couch, which, much to my surprise, turned out *not* to be perched over an invisible black hole where no one would ever see it again.

If You Can't Beat 'Em, Bribe 'Em

Hearing these stories, you might suspect I was quite a large child. But that wasn't true—pudgy would have described me well. I remember that by the end of fifth grade, I weighed a hundred pounds. But I also already had my period and was fully in puberty. At the time, and since my mother never weighed more than a hundred pounds in her life, this felt gargantuan to me. It wasn't until much later in life that a therapist told me something that rocked my world: "You know you were just growing, right?"

And, of course, the answer to that was no. I had absolutely no idea that adult women could acceptably weigh more than a hundred pounds or that my own weight gain was a natural part of growing up. By the time I was in late high school/college, I was a size 12/14, which is the American average,[4] but in my household might as well have been five times that.

Of course, I was too busy trying to lose weight to know anything about what was normal or okay or not. And my various attempts at weight loss kept me hooked because they were always successful—at least for a week or two. I'd lose a pound here, a couple of pounds there. Despite all the wishing and hoping imaginable, though, I was never one of those dramatic weight loss people.

My family environment ensured my focus on the external of my body, not the internal of how I felt. The only times I remember talking about what was going on inside me in relation to my body were when my parents were trying to cajole, motivate, or shame me into having more willpower. This focus on the external was writ large when they began to bribe me to lose weight.

In middle school, still young enough to be impressed by such things, I would get a new VHS tape of a movie I was interested in after I lost a pound (0.45 kg). This created something of a catch-22, though, because the more movies I got, the more I just wanted to stay in my room and watch them all (while eating, of course). However, I guess I really wanted to amass quite the collection because this is one of the times in my life that I lost the most weight—twenty pounds (9 kg). Twenty movies. Between that and the diet program, I'd imagine my folks were looking at about $75 a pound, which I'm sure they saw as a worthwhile investment.

And although it's been decades and I haven't owned a VHS player since the late '90s, it was only recently that I got rid of the last of those tapes.

Some things are just too hard-won.

Family, Love, and Mixed-Up "Good" Intentions

So far you've mostly heard, and will continue to hear, stories about how I relate to my body that involve my mom and not my dad. That's because my dad traveled Monday through Friday for all but the last couple years of my childhood.

I did have a few conversations with my dad about my weight and health over the years, though. Mostly, he tried to scare me into losing weight by telling me stories about how people in his family (like his dad) died young. The implication was always that if I didn't lose weight, I'd be counted among their number. It was only much later in life that I realized none of them died from anything weight-related at all and that his warnings came from his own projections and fears, not the actual reality of my body.

Mostly, my dad's perspective came through everything unsaid, or what my mom was somehow elected to convey to me, which is why you won't hear much about him.

Regardless of which parent conveyed the message to me on any given day, though, it wasn't coming solely from them—it was also wound up with the culture, both at large and in their own respective families.

For example, when I was a girl, my mom made me get on the scale in front of her on a near-weekly basis. The scale was in my parents' bathroom, which included one of those tiny rooms just for the toilet. For whatever inconceivable reason, the scale was in there. The room was painted a dark green, and it was insufferably hot. I can still feel the heat, flushed as I was with shame every time I had to go in there. I dreaded those weigh-ins, but it was hard to protest. If I did, it just added evidence in my mom's mind that she *had* to get me on the scale immediately. Clearly, if I was resisting, it was because I had something to hide. Our weekly weigh-ins continued like this for years—sometimes with cajoling, sometimes with distraction, sometimes with resistance—until I just couldn't take it anymore (and also had a teenager's attitude).

My exasperated mother could never understand my hesitation. I remember my dad even being on diets when I was growing up. I can still see the plates stacked high with bacon when he joined the low-carb craze in the early 2000s. And my mom simply weighed herself every day (so she thought our *weekly* check-ins were generous). Any rare time she noticed even a slight gain, she just restricted until it went away.

Easy breezy.

That seemingly simple equation never worked for me, though. So any time I had even a tiny gain, my mom would trot out her favorite "motivational" horror story: the fat people she knew and their miserable lives. She would give me the scoop on friends, neighbors, family members, people she saw on TV—anyone, really—all of whom were fat and supposedly hated their lives. She'd tell me about their struggles to lose weight: how they couldn't find relationships (or only got in bad ones); how much they loathed themselves; and how people were unlikely to want to know, love, or hire them because of their bodies. It wasn't right, she said, but it was reality. And she didn't want me to have to face it.

Of course, there is some truth to that. Fat discrimination is alive and well today, just as it was back then. But the bigger question I couldn't formulate then was why we had to accept it. I knew that dieting was as much a part of our family traditions as what we did on Christmas morning. I just never understood that it wasn't only my immediate family that was affected.

Until much later when I took a trip back home.

I went to visit my grandmother a while ago, and while I was with her, I thought a good deal about what she has taught me about loving my body.

She is the fiercest woman I know, and she's taught me a lot, but in this regard, my first, overwhelming thought was this: not too much.

My grandmother has Alzheimer's, and it's rare that she can remember what we just talked about half a minute ago, much less what I'm doing with my life these days.

What she remembers in fairly vivid detail, though, is her high school and college days—when she was a young woman who enjoyed hanging out with her friends and dating when she wasn't going to school, working several jobs, and taking care of her younger sister.

My grandmother had to grow up early. Really early.

She grew up in poverty, and she knew she wanted something different. So she started working—at multiple jobs, but also on reinventing herself. Both were partially because she wanted to and partially out of sheer necessity: She contributed to the family's bills from a very early age and often helped keep the lights on and food on the table.

She came from the "wrong side of the tracks" in many ways, but she wanted a different life. She wanted good manners, church, sobriety, a nice house, a presentable family. And how did women often get those things back then (and often still do today)? By disciplining their bodies to fit culturally determined norms.

As I sat looking at a photo album from my grandmother's youth, I noticed the commentary she'd written on each photo—who was who, where they had been. It was full of comments like "nice boy" beside an old beau—sweet stuff that made me smile, imagining her back then.

But then I increasingly noticed the comments she'd scratched in fiercely with a pen (so they couldn't be erased)—NO BEAUTY.

She'd written that on a photo of herself.

A gorgeous photo of herself.

My grandmother is, without a doubt, a beauty. She always has been and is no less so now in her eighties.

But what she isn't is sure of it. Because in the midst of the "NO BEAUTY" written comments was her live narration about how much she weighed during the various times of her life that were showcased in the album.

Her weight at different times in her life came up, I'd say, no less than ten times in the span of that short weekend visit. Both her weight now, as she turned to the side and proudly told us how small she is (because her Alzheimer's sometimes causes her to forget to eat), and her weight in high school, college, and during her pregnancies.

Her recollection was very precise—down to the exact pound. No guessing or struggling to remember necessary.

So of the increasingly few things my grandmother remembers with consistency and reliability these days, the one that is unfailing is her weight.

And she is a very, very thin woman; she always has been, though I hardly think this is by default. Her weight has clearly been a driving obsession her whole life, as it has been for every woman in our family (even if they wouldn't identify it that way), as it surely was for the women before her whom I didn't know.

As she continued her story, I exchanged sidelong glances with my husband when I could. When I did, I could feel such a clear understanding pass through both of us: "This explains so much." When we talked about it later, he agreed that's what he'd been thinking, too. I think he finally understood in that moment just how deep the food/weight/body obsession goes, and that it's definitely not just me.

Talking with my grandmother made it abundantly clear to me how our body insecurities are passed from generation to generation. For a long time, I thought this was something uniquely messed up about my own family, or that our obsession was stronger and worse than others'. And while of course all of our relationships to our bodies exist on a continuum, I now see so clearly how this issue is hardly one that finds its roots in my family. We're just a tiny limb branching off a much, much bigger tree that reaches into so many lives. And in my family, perhaps also as in yours, it's not too complicated to chart that reach.

I know I'm not alone in being raised in a family with a complicated relationship with food and bodies. Dieting and other efforts to change bodies that have been deemed unacceptable in one way or another are woven through many of our histories.

Knowing that my well-intentioned mother is reading this, I feel compelled to add that I know my parents meant well. Knowing that doesn't change the reality of my negative relationship with my body, but it does help me put in context that what I thought was my own individual "problem" actually extended far beyond me. It wasn't until I began to unpack how a need to control our bodies was an issue for many people in my family and beyond that I was able to look at my own history with more perspective.

Because what institutions like the diet industry want us to believe is that if we just work a little harder, we can achieve the societally acceptable body we want. Of course, all of this is rooted in all kinds of oppression that tell us what bodies are acceptable, when, and how. We often can't see that in our everyday lives, though, because the system is such that it blinds us to the collective and focuses us on the individual. So it makes sense that we all want to believe we'll be the exception to the rule and lose lots of weight and not gain it back (because most people can lose at least a little weight in the short term), though the odds are heavily stacked against us.[5] It's the perfect trap that ensures lifelong paying customers who then enlist their children in the same cycle and so on.

That my family, and maybe yours, got caught up in this is none too surprising. That's the whole point. And though my parents kept me in this system, it didn't start with them. They were simply trying to give me what society, and thus their families, said was a good life. It's just that that "good" life comes preloaded with self-hate and body hate. Individuals can't opt out of oppression. Becoming accepting of your own body doesn't mean that the culture will stop discriminating against fat bodies. What it can do, though, is give you the space to define yourself on your own terms.

Tallying the Numbers

Near the end of my decades-long standoff with my body, in a moment of sheer frustration, I decided to tally up the number of diets I'd been on in my life, expecting to come up with twenty, maybe thirty. So when I came up with sixty-five?

All I could do was cry.

When people say they've tried every diet out there, they're often *exaggerating*. But I'm pretty sure it's literally true for me, or pretty darn close.

And that's sixty-five *different* diets. I tried many of them multiple times. It's hard to say what's more staggering—the sheer number of weight loss techniques I've tried, or the amount of money I've spent on them. I've tried everything from hypnosis to a variety of diet drugs to weight loss teas to detoxes to fad diets and everything in between. I've never been able to get as clear a number on how much money my parents and I spent on weight loss endeavors over the years, but the number is easily in the thousands, and more likely tens of thousands.

And that number doesn't include the countless unpaid hours I spent researching, reading the latest diet book, coming up with elaborate change-my-life-on-Monday schemes, and more. Being on a diet was basically an unpaid (or worse—I had to pay for it myself), full-time job for me. So by the time I was in my late twenties, I was exhausted. I was going to graduate school full time while working four part-time jobs to make ends (barely) meet. I was wired all the time (I'm sure the weight loss pills I took intermittently didn't help), rarely sleeping more than a few hours.

And I was furious.

With myself.

Because I still couldn't manage to lose weight.

Despite (or, in retrospect, because of) all the diets I tried, the trend of my weight was always up, not down. By now, thanks to the addition of a diagnosis of polycystic ovarian syndrome, which affects hormone levels and the body's ability to process blood sugar, I was up to a size 20 and couldn't figure out where I kept going "wrong." I was in the process of finishing a second master's degree. I had a wonderful husband and a great relationship with him. I had friends who had my back and vice versa. My two adorable dogs made me laugh every day.

So how on Earth could I be so successful in every other arena of my life but keep failing so miserably at this one?!

I was miserably unhappy, I didn't get it, and I felt like an utter failure.

But soon, the truth began to dawn on me.

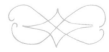

MAY I
appreciate
MY BODY
a little more
IN
this moment

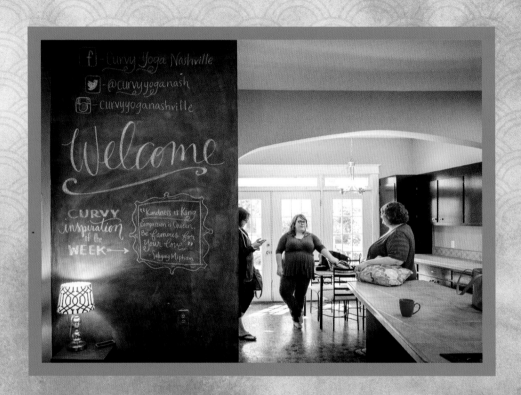

Presence

Did You Know You Have to Know Your Body Before Accepting It? Me, Neither.

What I discovered is that in order to get started with changing my relationship with my body, I first had to be present in and with it—actually know what it was feeling in the moment. Wild, I know.

In order to be more present with my body, I first had to unpack the times I'd had my fingers in my ears and ignored it. I needed to do that to remind myself that my body wasn't a dull lump that never had anything to say, as I'd always suspected, but rather that I just hadn't yet become fluent in its language.

One of the first memories that came to mind along those lines was when I was in my mid-twenties. My maternal grandfather was dying of the same cancer my dad had just been diagnosed with months before; the present and future were intertwined in a painful way.

At the same time, I was convinced that I was on the verge of having a heart attack. This fear didn't come out of nowhere: My paternal grandfather had died of one (though that was related to complications from surgery due to an accident), and my dad lived in fear of one, so that fear seeped into me. I went to the doctor, and after listening to my heart and not finding anything, he asked me what was going on in my life. What stress I was facing. Offhandedly, I mentioned what was going on with my grandfather and my dad. But this isn't about that, I said—this is an actual physical pain. "I have that feeling they always mention of an elephant sitting on my chest, and that doesn't seem right."

He listened to my heart again and told me he was going to keep an eye on it and that I should come back if it didn't improve. I waited an excruciating week, sure I'd die at any moment but more afraid of being seen as a hypochondriac, and then I returned. I told him, with more than a little desperation, that nothing had changed. That, if anything, I was worse.

Probably more to protect himself than anything, he sent me for a test. Relieved, I submitted to the scan, grateful to now know what was wrong with me. Glad to catch it before it was too late. Imagining what people would say at my funeral if it *was* already too late.

A short while later, the doctor came back to report that I was fine. The test didn't show any problems, and I was good to go. He gently mentioned that grief and stress could cause physical sensations. I felt chastened but also surprised and kind of pissed.

Why couldn't I just be having a heart attack? That, I'd know how to deal with. That, someone else could manage.

I wish I could say this was a breakthrough moment when everything changed and suddenly I listened to and was present with my body. But you probably already know me well enough by now to know that's not true.

When Things Started to Change

Because while the moment with the doctor was an eye-opening one, it didn't stay with me as much as you might suspect. For one thing, that remained a stressful time in my life for quite a while, and I was too caught up in all that for it to stick with me. Also, I could only truly understand how much my body was speaking to me when I felt it myself, not just when someone else told me about it.

Around this same time, I'd started practicing hot yoga with a man with endless energy, who had to have been in his seventies at minimum, and whom I never saw wear anything but tiny shorts.

I was an unlikely student for him.

But the thought of potential weight loss from the heat drew me in. I'd been practicing yoga for over five years at that point, but never in a hot room, as that had only recently started to become popular. During my first class, I thought I might pass out. I had to lie down on the floor several times and breathe. I'd never breathed in what felt like fire before, but that's how hot the air was in this room.

Despite this (or perhaps because of it, due to my undying belief at the time in "No pain, no gain"), I went back. And the next time, I only had to lie down a couple times. The next time after that, only once. And so on. Each time I went to class, I left feeling a little more determined to return.

Then, one day, the unimaginable happened. I went to an afternoon class that was never very full. After all, only students and a handful of other people are available to attend a yoga class at that time. So for a few minutes, it was just me and my teacher. But then I heard the bell attached to the door indicating that some other people had arrived. I'd chosen a spot in the middle row, far-right side of the room and was doing some casual stretches, waiting for class to begin. Then in came ten bustling, chattering young women. They all had a similar, fit look, and it was easy to tell they knew each other well.

Soon enough, our teacher started class and welcomed the local university women's soccer team. That's right: It was my teacher, ten athletes, and me. I was only a few years older than they were at best, but I felt that we couldn't be more different.

Great.

As class started, I considered my escape route. I was already close to the door, so maybe I could just slip out. Pretend that I forgot a grad school emergency (as though that's a thing). Fake a fainting spell (which wasn't entirely out of the realm of possibility in that hot room). Before I knew it, though, I'd spent too long hatching schemes to get away with any of them. I was stuck.

My strategy was to point my face toward the mirror but avoid my own eye contact. There was no *way* I wanted to see how those other women were looking at me, or how they looked in their poses. There I was, trying to keep my belly from popping out of my shirt and trying to pretend that I had the confidence to pull off the tight workout clothing I was sporting because nothing else really works in the hot room. And there they were, svelte and toned, looking like that workout clothing was made with them in mind. I silently cursed both them and myself, furious at how easily this was all going to come to them.

Except, it didn't.

At all.

These women were thin and fit, but they weren't particularly flexible. They also weren't particularly coordinated; perhaps they had overworked their hand/eye coordination in one direction so much that it was underdeveloped in others.

I sort of noticed they were having a hard time of it, but I was still mostly focused on just doing my thing and pretending that no one else was there to fully register it. Because of that, I couldn't focus on much more than my own experience, what was happening in my body. Finally, we made it to the floor portion of the class, and we were doing one of my favorite things: side splits. We'd get in there from a standing wide-legged forward bend, then with our hands on the floor, we'd start walking our legs wider and wider, until maybe, just maybe, our pelvises would come to the floor.

This pose didn't come naturally to me—far from it. In fact, the first time I tried it, I think I pulled about thirteen muscles in my exuberance to get to the floor no matter what. Once I recovered, I realized that my mind wasn't going to help me learn my boundaries—when to back off and when to try a new challenge. But I had a hunch that my body might, seeing that it was the only resource still available that I hadn't tried. Over time, through going slowly and beginning to be present with and learn my body's signals of what was possible (or not), I slowly became comfortable in the pose.

So during this particular class, I couldn't have been more surprised when I heard the magic words: "See what Anna is doing over there? Do it like that."

For a second, I forgot my own name. *See what Anna is doing? Who's that? Is there another Anna in here?* And then I looked over and saw it: All eyes were on me. With shock, I caught my teacher's eye, and he gave me a secret smile. From my unwitting demonstration, the women registered the part of the pose they were missing, and the rest of the class carried on as usual.

When I left class, the soccer gals were chatting with the teacher, so I slipped out the door. The next time I saw him a few days later, though, he smiled widely. "I just loved the other day, didn't you?"

I'm not sure I've ever had a prouder moment in my life.

Someone was proud of me for showing up in my body, *this* body, and doing my thing. And, of course, that person was my teacher.

But even more important, that person was also me.

Because what I'd been able to illustrate to my fellow classmates that day had nothing to do with my weight, which hadn't changed, or the fact that I was easily ten sizes bigger than the rest of them, at minimum.

Rather, it had to do with me. Though I hadn't appreciated the soccer team's attention at the time or the hot mess I'd thought I was on the mat, this moment showed me something concrete (because subtlety so wasn't the name of my game) about my ability to be present in my body and respond to it: that it *was* possible after all, and that yoga was playing a big part.

You Do Yoga?

I didn't come to yoga originally to accept my body. Quite the opposite. I started it when I was eighteen to reduce pain from my then-chronic migraines and, well, to lose weight. It just seemed obvious that if I kept practicing, it would only be a matter of time until I looked like the people who led the tapes I practiced with. Those folks were lean and lithe, and the yoga poses all seemed to be cheerfully effortless for them. I got into yoga before there was much that was specifically weight-loss focused, so I picked up most of my "yoga = perfect body" messages through osmosis (and, of course, projections and desires from all my past weight loss endeavors).

Yoga classes weren't on every corner in the late '90s, as they are now, so I didn't start practicing in classes for a few years because there weren't any where I lived at the time. My first in-person yoga teacher was a woman who literally had blue hair and had to have at least been in her eighties. I was the youngest person there by a minimum of four decades, and we didn't have yoga mats or props. We practiced in a local community center on those thick mats (also blue) they have in gyms. I don't know what kept me, a highly self-conscious, curvy, barely twenty-something going back, but I did.

In taking up yoga, I was engaging for the first time in a movement practice for reasons other than solely weight loss. Up until then, any exercise I'd undertaken had been purely to discipline my body, to punish myself for my size. I even joined the girls' golf team at my high school and played on the backup team for three years for that reason. Me! Golf! (And in case you're wondering if I was any good at it, the answer is: not at all.)

So when I found something that I kind of loved? I wanted to do it all the time! After all those years of forcing myself to do exercise that I didn't like or kind of liked but that couldn't stop me from thinking about how many calories I was burning the whole time, thus ruining it, I was delightfully surprised to find something different in yoga. I'd never known I could look forward to moving my body; in fact, I'd assumed that no one could, that some people were just better at doing it out of obligation.

Because of this radical new relationship to movement I'd found via yoga, I was *minutely* less insistent about losing weight through it. In the past, when I was on the treadmill, you'd better believe I was counting out every painstakingly burned calorie. Why else was I there, walking all those miles to nowhere, next to "Sprinty Sprinterson" on the treadmill beside me? But with yoga, while part of me assumed I would lose weight just based on the other yogis I saw, I didn't care about it *quite* as much—which is to say, I still *really* cared about it.

But I'd also started to care about other things, too, like that glowy feeling after *Savasana* (the final relaxation pose of many yoga classes) or the relief of the first deep breath to start class. The road to getting present with my body through yoga didn't start with angels singing or deep flashes of insight into the nature of reality. Instead, it started with the most fleeting, easy-to-catch moments of just feeling good: nothing more complex, or profound, than that. Being present with my body was a doorway into a deeper relationship with myself that I didn't even realize I was walking through. All I knew was that I felt something and I wanted to keep feeling it.

Wearing Me Down

When I look back, I can see so many times in my life when my body was trying to get my attention but I wasn't present enough to be able to listen: during that weight loss meeting in middle school when all I wanted to do was get the heck out of there, during my weekly weigh-ins when I'd get so hot I'd want to pass out, when I thought I was having a heart attack but I was really just sad, and so many others.

When all those things were happening, though, I couldn't see them as times that my body was speaking to me. I don't know that I saw them as anything at all, except what we've already talked about—further evidence of my body's inability to get with the program and do what I wanted it to do. I was too busy trying to avoid, ignore, or otherwise get rid of the uncomfortable feelings those episodes brought up to look any deeper.

And I also didn't have the knowledge or skills to look deeper until much later in my life.

I believe that starting to reflect on times when your body has indeed been speaking to you is one way the process of body acceptance begins. Taking note of those moments reminds you that you already have a relationship with your body, even if it hasn't felt like it for a very long time—or ever.

In addition, recalling times your body has been speaking in the past helps you start identifying clues as to when it's talking today. With the examples I've shared with you so far, some of my own signs have come up: feeling flushed; being anxious; wanting to crawl out of my skin or disappear; hiding, hating, and berating myself. When I feel these things today, they make me stop and think: "What else is going on here?" Because now I know that these feelings are reactions to something deeper that is going on, not evidence of how I'm terrible and need a new body, as I'd always thought.

Of course, this all starts with what we've been talking about—getting present with your body. I know that word is a little overused in some circles today, but it's what I've found to be the best way to describe how you actually get started with accepting your body. Because that process doesn't start with your mind (despite how many of us might like to *think* our way there). It starts in your body, with something as simple as feeling your feet on the floor or your bum on the chair seat. Once you do that, you shift into a body-led place that can guide you into the next part of this practice: getting curious.

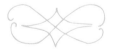

PRACTICES

From here on out, I'm going to offer you a few simple practices in each chapter that have helped me on my own journey and that I've seen support my yoga students as well. They're all designed to facilitate the process of using yoga as a tool for body acceptance. You can experiment with these however you like—trying them before moving on to the next chapter or bookmarking them for later. The main thing I want you to know is that you can always come back to these anytime you feel that you need a little encouragement and a reminder that this path and process are indeed possible for you. You can come back to these as often as you need. They're absolutely intended to be practices that help you build, and later sustain, a relationship with your body over time, not one-and-done techniques to "fix" you instantaneously (because you don't need fixing).

If you'd like audio versions of the practices, visit www.curvyyoga .com/book.

Presence on the Yoga Mat

One of the ways to practice presence is directly on your yoga mat. Many yoga classes start with a form of being present, or centering. That time often includes getting your body aligned and doing some breath work.

One way you can do this on your own is by noticing where you're in contact with your yoga mat. For example, if you're seated on a blanket, move your attention to your feet and just simply note where your feet are in contact with the floor. There's nothing to change (unless you need to in order to be more comfortable). You can move up your body from there and note where your legs are in contact with your mat/blanket, as well as your bum. You might then see if it's possible to lengthen your spine at all. From there, take a few deep breaths.

This might sound so simple as to not warrant its own part of our practice, but it's actually the ground of it all. Many of us have been told that it's not okay to inhabit our bodies for many different reasons. So when we try it (with support from others as needed, particularly if there's trauma in your background), we build our ability to do so in the future with more ease. This matters because it's very difficult—I'd even venture to say impossible—to have a relationship with your body without knowing what it feels like.

Presence Off the Yoga Mat

You can also engage the same process as above off your yoga mat. I like to do the practice—presence, get curious, challenge, and affirm—at natural transition times in the day. For example, one time I find this works well for me is when I wake up in the morning. Before I get up, I take a moment to notice (from feet to head) where I'm in contact with the bed. That helps me transition from sleeping to waking and also helps me start the day by connecting with my body. I might also do this at lunch time, after work, and before going to bed. When you do it doesn't matter; finding times that work for you and that are easy enough for you to remember is what matters.

Body Check-In

If you want to get curious about what's going on in your body right here, right now, you can. As in, you can literally do it right this minute. I hate it when these types of exercises tell you to read it, then set your book down and do it. Instead, we're just going to do it together, right now. So just as you're reading here, start to soften your gaze on this book and expand your peripheral vision. There's nothing for you to do or achieve except noticing what's around you. Oftentimes, sharpening your attention on your external environment helps you settle into awareness, which you can then turn toward your internal environment with a bit more ease.

Now tune into pressure: Notice where you're in contact with whatever you're sitting, standing, or lying on. Are you shifted more to one side of your body than the other? What is your back in contact with, if anything? What's the temperature of what you're in contact with? There's absolutely nothing for you to change right now, though if you find something that would allow you to sit/stand/lie more comfortably, go ahead and do that.

Take three deep breaths, allowing each one to deepen any amount more than the one before. You can do this as you continue reading, or just pause at the end of this sentence until you're done, then continue from there.

Now turn your attention to your feet: First just observe whatever comes into your field of awareness. This could be their position in space, what they're in contact with, how they feel, their temperature, and so on. Again, there is no "right" answer here. Whatever you observe is exactly what you're looking for. In fact, even if you don't notice a thing, that's also the kind of information you're looking for. It's all just what's happening now, and not knowing is also something that's happening. As above, if you find any little shifts or adjustments you'd like to make to be more comfortable, make those movements in the feet.

Let's continue this process, now moving to the hips. Begin by observing whatever you can about the hips, perhaps even using some of your deep breaths from before to drop into a place where you can listen inside. Then make any refinements to your position that may present themselves (including none!).

Now do the same for your shoulders, following the same process we've been doing, but on your own, allowing the end of this sentence and paragraph to give you time before you move on.

Finally, expand your awareness through your whole body and ask yourself this question: "If I could name how I'm feeling in one word, what would it be?" Simply note whatever arises, and don't get hung up on the one-word thing. That can be a way to simplify, but if you come up with two words or two paragraphs, it really doesn't matter. Again, it's all information about what's going on inside you, and that's what we want.

Just a quick word for any self-doubters out there (raising my hand!): If you did this exercise, got a word, and thought something to the effect of "This?! I'm not feeling this! I'm feeling that!" or "That can't be right!" or "I can't even tell how I feel; I'm doomed!," don't worry. You're not alone. In fact, I think you're in the majority, and

I've been right there with you for most of my life. Most of us have not been taught to notice, much less trust, the way we're feeling. Most of us have been told, starting in childhood, that we're not feeling what we're actually feeling. Or not to feel the way we're feeling and instead to "cooperate," "be quiet," or "stop crying." Uncertainty about how you're feeling isn't a sign of failure. It's a sign of deep engagement in the process. Keep going! This is a skill you can build, just like a muscle.

So now what do you do with this information about how you're feeling? Well, that depends on what you found out. If you discovered that one of your needs is unmet—say, you're hungry, thirsty, tired, have to go to the bathroom, or the like—then see what you can do to meet that need right now in a doable way. For example, if you're tired but reading this on the train on your way to work, you may not be able to get off and go home for a nap. But what *could* you do right now? Stand up? Reach your arms overhead? Yawn? Put on some good music when you get off and walk into work? This is where you get to start experimenting and see just how clever—and simple—you can make things to build trust with yourself so that you can, indeed, meet your own needs and feel your feelings.

It's from this place of growing self-trust, no matter how minuscule it may seem, that you can begin to enter into a new paradigm and relationship with your body.

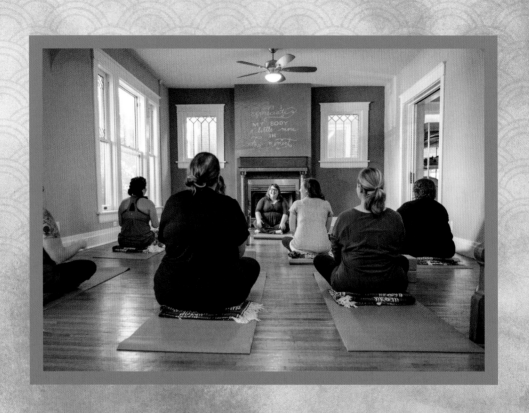

Get Curious:

Finding the Voices in Your Head That You Can Trust

One of the ways I started to get curious about my body's signs was by noticing how my body feels in a given moment. I started doing this first on my yoga mat because it turned out that I'd been getting tiny clues to the answer in every yoga class I'd ever attended. It just wasn't until later that I realized every time my yoga teacher asked me to do something, like feel what was going on in my body, that she meant it literally.

Because, though I enjoyed the movements of yoga when I first started practicing, I had no idea what I was feeling in my body in any concrete way. I guessed things were happening, mostly because my teacher said so, but I didn't really know what they were for me.

For example, in class, my teacher would say something like "Notice what's going on with your baby toe in this pose," and I'd just inwardly smile. I thought this was just yoga-teacher-speak, the stuff of frilly metaphors like "Blossom your buttocks," "Send energy shooting out your fingers," or other yoga-isms. I truly didn't believe anyone felt any of those things, even the more concrete ones; I just thought they were nice things to say.

It wasn't until one class a few years in that I finally heard my teacher when she said, "Feel what's happening in your baby toe." I mean, my ears had heard her say it many times in the past. But I'd never heard it—much less felt it—in my body until that moment.

And when it happened, it kinda freaked me out.

I had expected to find, as I had so many other times, nothing. Honestly, I'd all but tuned that talk out, so meaningless did it seem to me. After so many years of quashing my body's signals in favor of following the rules of my latest diet, it had become all but impossible for me to notice anything going on with my body. But this time, as my inner awareness woke up, I felt the uniquely squishy yet firm sensation of the mat underneath my baby toe. And I noticed how the inside of my toe was pressed down more than the outside, telling me I wasn't fully engaging my whole foot in the pose.

I couldn't believe it.

In fact, I didn't believe it—until I started trying it with my other foot, then other body parts. As I engaged in this inner observation, I felt tears come to my eyes. I'd found a whole part of myself that I hadn't even known was missing.

Which was, of course, my whole body.

I found a way to listen to my body, which before this had only been theoretical, because of how yoga asked me to notice what was going on in what turned out to be concrete detail. There was something about being asked to notice a specific body part, bodily action, or breath in a particular movement that brought listening to my body into stark relief. That attention to detail gave me the anchor and space I needed to get curious about what else might be happening in this body of mine.

I've found that curiosity is such an important factor in building your body awareness, that without it, learning to listen to and accept your body largely stays in the realm of seems-like-a-good-idea but isn't actually possible or practical. Curiosity, though, brings us into a process, a dialogue with our body where we can move into an open place of wonder—what's happening here?— rather than imposing our will as many of our old habits try to enforce.

Curiosity has an inherently light and playful way about it that has nothing to do with getting anything right or wrong. It would never say, "What's wrong with you?"/"Why aren't you in better tune with your body?"/"You'll never get anything right," as many of the voices do from our trying-to-change-our-body days. Instead, it says without judgment, "Hmm . . . what is my body telling me?" There is such freedom in this shift from control and/or disconnection to curiosity because it sees in grays, not just black and white.

Getting curious brings you into the present moment with your body by actually engaging it in a dialogue. This is essential because when you're in the current truth of your embodied experience, the negative voices in your head have less room than they used to. From that place of neutral awareness, you can remind yourself that your inner critic's voice isn't the only one that counts and find a way to move forward.

How Curiosity Led Me to Become a Yoga Teacher

Curiosity is actually what led me to become a yoga teacher (because as I mentioned, this is the absolute last thing I ever thought I'd be doing with my life). For years and years I'd practiced in classes where the teachers were generally nice enough but mostly ignored me, never offering suggestions on how to make the practice work for my body when I was clearly struggling.

I just kept assuming I'd really *get* yoga and be able to implement all the teacher's instructions once I finally lost all the weight I wanted to. I figured that must be what I needed since (1) I was almost always the biggest person in the room and (2) the teachers never suggested that anyone might be facing the challenges I was, so I concluded that the problem must be me.

Over time, though, and once my body acceptance journey had started, I had a thought that changed my life: "What if my body isn't the problem? What if the problem is just that my teachers never learned how to teach bodies like mine?" Not only was "What if my body *isn't* a problem?" a total inner revolution (seriously; I recommend all of us ask ourselves this anytime we start thinking something is a problem with our body, whether yoga-related or not), the teaching question freed me to get curious. Was it really that simple?

What I found was that my instinct was right: Most teachers were learning very little to nothing in their training about working with curvy bodies. And with that, the idea of becoming a teacher began percolating in my mind. Because, to me, it just seemed like common sense: The majority of people do not live in thin, fit, flexible, able bodies, so by not learning how to teach those bodies, yoga teachers were leaving far too many people out of the practice who could benefit from it. And since I couldn't find the resources I'd been looking for, I thought I'd see what I could do to create some, particularly around how yoga can work as a tool for body acceptance.

At the time, I was teaching English and had been practicing yoga for almost a decade. Since I knew I liked teaching and yoga, I guessed I might also like teaching yoga. But unlike today when it's much easier to find a yoga teacher–training program, I spent the next couple years looking and never finding one.

So when one did finally come to town, at the studio where I practiced, I took it as a sign. But I was still completely unsure if I could do it, if I should do it, and, even more importantly, if I would get accepted. So one day after class, I snuck the info flyer into my bag and took it home with me.

Once I was home I reviewed the information on the flyer and corresponding website. You had to fill out an application and meet with one of the teachers to join, the thought of which made me want to throw up. But something kept prodding me along, and I continued responding, mostly because I also kept telling myself all I was doing was taking one more step and that I didn't actually have to go through with it.

On the day I went to the interview with the teacher, I came *this close* to not leaving my house at all. Then once I got in my car, I drove past the studio and circled the block before finally pulling into the parking lot. Once in the parking lot, I seriously considered leaving, but I was afraid it was too late because the parking lot was gravel and I could tell that the teacher was inside and would have heard me; we were the only two people there. When I walked up to the door, I almost passed out from nerves. And when we sat down to talk, I mostly just listened, wide-eyed, waiting for the moment she'd tell me I should wait until I lost some weight to participate. I even made it easy for her to do so, giving her an out by suggesting I thought it might be a problem myself.

But as fate would have it, she didn't say that. She said she was excited to have me in the program. So, elated (if the meaning of that is terrified), I paid my deposit and joined.

Getting curious is the next step in our practice after being present, because we can't move forward until we know where we are, and that often involves asking ourselves directly. Of course, noticing can take many different forms. For the rest of this chapter, let's look at some of the ways it shows up both on and off the yoga mat to spark some ideas about what you might start to notice in your own body and life.

There were several months between signing up and the program starting, and I spent that time in a mix of feeling delighted and feeling that I should definitely drop out. I started practicing more and more often, determined not to be the big girl in class who couldn't do what everyone else could.

As the time for the start of the program drew closer, I started to breathe just a *little* easier, feeling that now I'd committed myself and it was too late to change my mind. There was just one problem: I ended up breaking my ankle the weekend before the teacher-training program was to begin.

So, yes, my worst nightmare had come true: I was literally the big girl sitting out in the back of the room while everyone else did the yoga practice.

I could have died.

What kept me going, though I considered dropping out several times, and what eventually made me teach my first class, though I was petrified, was my instinct that I couldn't be the only person in the whole wide world who'd been looking for a body-affirming yoga class. I just knew there had to be at least a *couple* of other people out there who wanted to connect with their body through yoga, and I wanted to find them.

Lo and behold, as I started teaching and talking with people all over the world, I discovered how not alone I was in wanting to know and connect with my own body as it was. There are so many of us! And what I've found over the years of talking with folks is that curiosity was key for them, too.

Question Your Body

Curiosity takes many different forms in relation to your practice. If you're new to noticing what's going on with your body, or even if you're not and you want to deepen your current capacity, it starts and continues with coming back to noticing what's going on.

With noticing, we have to be careful not to make the mistake of letting ourselves think it's something that works within a success/failure paradigm. It's very tempting to go there because most of us know that well, but we can't let ourselves because curiosity exists outside of success or failure. It works like the tides—in its own ebbing and flowing relationship with its own moon, which is you and your experiences in your body.

If this all feels a bit confusing, don't worry—yoga gives us a way in. It not only gives you an opportunity to practice the inner awareness necessary for body acceptance, it also gives you some frameworks to do that. One of those frameworks is called the *koshas*. The *koshas* are the layers (also translated as "sheaths") of our body and being, and they give you a way to think about *how* yoga works on and in you. I don't know about you, but I can use all the help I can get to make body acceptance a practical, concrete part of my life, not just a pie-in-the-sky abstract concept.

I like to think of the *koshas* like nesting dolls. Each of the five layers is often referred to as a body, but that doesn't mean you have five different bodies. That terminology just helps us think about the different layers of our being in both discrete and interconnected ways.

Here's what they are:

ANNAMAYA KOSHA This is your physical body, the outer layer. It's often the first door into this journey of yoga, happening through the yoga poses (this is what I was noticing that time I first felt my baby toe on the mat), and then you continue on from there. Not that you stop working with this one, though; that's part of the beauty of how this all works. It's a very reciprocal process.

PRANAMAYA KOSHA This is your energy body (*prana* means "energy"). The easiest way for you to connect with this is usually through your breath, which can be a bridge that helps you connect mind and body.

MANOMAYA KOSHA This is your mental/emotional body. *Mano* means "mind," so this is where you process thoughts and feelings. It's here that your practice increases your awareness of your thoughts and also shifts your thought patterns over time.

VIJNANAMAYA KOSHA This is your subtle body, inner wisdom. As you continue through the *koshas,* using the ones that came before to clear the way, you can receive these messages from your body, heart, and soul more and more clearly.

ANANDAMAYA KOSHA This is the bliss body. How great is that?! This isn't necessarily the happy bliss state we think of, but more a sense of oneness. Though some people think of this as something developed only through something like enlightenment, I like to think of it as wholeness or integration—less something you achieve and more something you feel your way into, even in the most fleeting of moments.

While none of the *koshas* are destinations or clear demarcations ("Oh, today I finally accessed my *anandamaya kosha*!"), they do give you one way to understand the process that's unfolding both on and off your yoga mat.

For example, sometimes people will say while in a yoga pose that they don't "feel it." What that usually means is they're not finding a physical stretch. While it's possible that they may just need some refining in their alignment, it's also important to note that where the pose may be working with them more on that particular day is with their breath (*pranamaya kosha*), or it may be helping them quiet their mind (*manomaya kosha*); it could also be increasing their awareness of what's going on inside their body (*vijnanamaya kosha*).

The *koshas* can both deepen your awareness of how yoga works and give you some ways into deeper body acceptance by showing you that there are more doorways in than just the physical body. Because sometimes, if connecting with the physical body isn't working for you in any given moment, turning to the breath or noticing your feeling state may very well be what helps you shift to a deeper understanding of your body in the moment.

The *koshas* can also help you understand why and how yoga is such a powerful tool for body acceptance. The framework itself really lays it out for us—first we connect with our physical body. Then, as we become more comfortable and familiar with that, our inner awareness develops, and we might be able to start noticing how we feel, or the negative thoughts we have about our body that aren't helping us. As our awareness grows, so does our capacity to take action because we finally know what's been going on all along, which gives us insight into how we might want to move forward.

If you want to practice noticing the different layers of your body and being on your mat, begin with being present, as discussed in the previous chapter. See what and how much you can identify happening in your body (there's more on this in the practices at the end of this chapter). Observing the physical body might be enough for today. But whenever you want to extend that process, you can continue from the physical body to the breath. Without changing the pacing or phrasing of your natural breath, begin to notice: Where do you feel the breath moving in your body? Some people notice it more at the nostrils— entering and exiting. Other people connect better through the rise and fall of their chest or belly. Wherever it's easiest for you to notice is the right place for you. As you continue to breathe, observe with gentle curiosity the length of your inhale compared to your exhale. For most people, there is a difference. Again, there is nothing to change here. You're just becoming acquainted with your own breath.

After some breath observation, you could then turn your attention to how you're feeling. Ask yourself: In one word or short phrase, how would I describe what I'm feeling right now? This simple exercise is a great way to start being more specific with yourself about how you feel—especially if you've tried something like this in the past and found it difficult or impossible. Once you name your current feeling, see if there's any place it's living in your body. And if that sounds like a wild question, no worries. All you have to do is pose the question and see what happens. Nothing might happen at all. But you might also be surprised to find that your body does, indeed, have an answer for you once the question is asked. For example, the word you might have come up with when asking your body how it's feeling is stressed, and when you ask where it lives, you might find the answer is in your shoulders, jaw, or wherever you tend to hold tension. When something like that presents itself, you have the opportunity to shift it, by relaxing your shoulders or whatever makes sense for you. Continue to stay with that feeling and physical location for a minute or so and see what happens. Very often, our feeling state shifts much more quickly than we tend to think it will in our everyday life. Yoga can be a wonderful way to further notice and affirm this process, building our resilience so we remember it later, off the mat, when we feel overwhelmed by emotion.

Now that we've moved through the physical body, breath, and feelings, it's possible to drop into your inner wisdom. Ask yourself: "What do I need to know or remember right now?" Again, who knows if an answer will arise today? It may or may not. What matters more is that you pose the question with openness and see what happens. As this question is asked on a regular basis, the body begins to realize that you're listening and those messages may appear (and this could also happen on your first day of asking—it's different for everyone).

From here, expand your awareness through your whole body, integrating body, breath, feeling, and subtle body. This feeling of oneness is what some might call the "bliss body."

Of course, experiencing these layers of being isn't always as straightforward as I just described. It can be—certainly many yoga classes or guided meditations follow a similar trajectory—but not always (and rarely in everyday life). They can also be experienced in a different order, simultaneously, one but not others, and so on. The main thing I hope you take away here is that this is a way to start getting curious about the signals your body is sending, allowing you to respond. And if connecting with one part or layer of your body/being is challenging, you can try another. Over time, you'll begin to create your own custom blend of what helps you connect with your body best.

Get Curious about Your Feelings

As the *koshas* showed us, the body includes more than physical sensation; it also includes our thoughts and feelings. It's important to note that yoga is not, as it is often misunderstood to be, a way to avoid or transcend your feelings. It's not about becoming so chill that you never feel anything again: That's becoming a zombie, not a yogi. Yoga is often translated as "yoke" or "union." Either way, the meaning is clear—connection, not disconnection; noticing, not oblivion; awareness, not living in a dream. The goal isn't to feel less, or to feel nothing. The goal is to feel what you're feeling. Because it's only when you feel your feelings that you don't stay stuck in, hide from, or obsess over them.

Let's take how you feel about your body as an example. Like I mentioned, for years I covered over and ignored how I felt both in and about my body. But as we've discussed, that hardly helped. I deeply believe that ignoring those feelings is what kept me trapped in the cycle of yo-yo dieting and body hate for longer than was necessary. The more I tried to hide it with yet another diet, the worse I felt. I think I feared that if I actually let it come to the surface, it would swallow me whole.

For a very, very long time, my default reaction to just about every feeling I had was repression. Like many people, I recognize this is due to some personal blend of life's difficulties, hating my body, and what was available to me at the time. If I'd grown up in a family of drinkers or drug users, perhaps I would have turned to those things. But I only had two readily available options to help me cope with life: food and forgetting.

And for me, the two are related. Whenever anything hard happened to me, I would disassociate, or leave my body, and forget . . . well, pretty much everything. And thanks to almost always being deprived due to my latest diet, as well as complicated relationships with food abounding in my family, I also turned to food, including binge eating. Bingeing has its own particular blackout quality to it, so between that, dieting, and disassociating, I was very rarely in my body. All of those behaviors happened unconsciously, which meant that since I didn't knowingly turn them on, I also didn't know how to turn them off. For much of my life, I didn't even know that they were on at all; I thought that's just how my life was. Both bingeing/dieting and forgetting laid the groundwork of disembodiment for me—not knowing how I felt—or that I felt anything at all.

What happened when I started to feel my feelings thanks to yoga wasn't that it swallowed me whole. Instead, when I started to feel, I could see a feeling for what it was—"Oh, this is a feeling." Knowing I was feeling something rather than believing the story that feeling generated in me was freeing. For example, rather than hiding inside all day because I couldn't bear going out due to what I thought was the truth of my hideous body, I began to feel the bodily sensations underneath those thoughts and realize "Oh, I'm feeling vulnerable." Or "Wow, I'm really tired." There was something so helpful about feeling the bodily sensation and naming it because it brought me out of my stories and into what was actually happening in my body in real time, which is a much more empowering place from which to operate.

Get Curious about Your Breath

One of the things that helps me begin to notice bodily sensation and how I feel is my breath. The breath is what ties together the often-discussed yet often-misunderstood mind-body connection. Because the mind and body *are* already connected, but since we're human, we forget and need reminders.

"Count your inhale: 1, 2, 3 . . . until you get to the top," a well-known but new to me teacher coaxed. "Exhale out one beat longer, then retain the breath. Hoooooooooold. Hold . . . Begin again."

I'd done this particular practice many times before, maybe a hundred, maybe a thousand. But this day I was doing it for the first time since my dad had died about five months earlier. As I lay back, held my breath, and felt my desire for an inhale rise, everything went dark. I felt as if I had slipped through some hole in time and I was right back there with him as he lay dying. That I was him. That I was somehow dying his death and dying my own death and also still alive. Maybe. I was still alive, right? In that moment, I couldn't have told you for sure.

As I lay at the front of the class, wedged between another student and the teacher of this class, not an inch (2.5 cm) between any mat in the room or any way to escape, all I could do was breathe at my own pace. There was no way for me to leave the room, though I wanted to, so I just had to stay there and feel everything that was happening in the present moment, which is the only place the breath ever exists.

Before that moment, even after having practiced yoga for a dozen years and taught for a few, I'd never *really* felt the potency of my own breath. I mean, sure, I'd understood it on an abstract level. I'd heard yoga people say that it's a portal to our *prana*, or life-force energy. But I didn't *get* it—until then.

What I glimpsed in that moment is how the breath integrates the functions of the whole body. When I dropped my attention from everyday concerns and focused on my breath, my current embodied experience of grief was immediately there, as though it had been waiting for me to notice it for months—which it surely had been.

Though the breath is our constant companion through this life, even when labored or halting, becoming aware of it is slow and subtle work. You know how sometimes when you haven't seen a friend for a while, you run into her and you can tell something about her is different, but you have no idea what it is? "I cut eight inches (20.5 cm) off my hair," she exclaims. Or, "I got new glasses!" "Yes!" you sigh, as though you'd noticed it yourself. New glasses—that's it. Or as it sometimes happens for me, someone else has this insight. I hadn't observed a physical difference, but when someone else calls it out, it's clear. How could I have missed something so seemingly obvious?

We often can't see what's right in front of us. Much less what is inside us. The way we begin to get curious about the breath is to approach it with an attitude of playfulness. When your yoga teacher asks you to inhale on a particular movement and exhale during another one, let that be a suggestion and not a command. One of the ways to know more about your own breath is to observe your own patterns. How does an inhale feel when you reach your arms overhead? What about when you do the same thing on an exhale? When do you feel a breath behind? Or ahead? What happens to your breath during *Savasana* (the final relaxation pose of most yoga classes)? Or what about while reading a stressful email? Or finding yourself in a negative body image moment?

As I deepened my relationship with my breath, I began to catch glimpses of it during everyday life. And what I noticed is this: I hold my breath. Constantly. This pattern followed me both on and off the yoga mat. What's interesting is how the things we get curious about in our bodies can teach us about other parts of our lives, too. As I noticed my pattern of holding my breath, I began to make some associations. For example, any time I found myself holding my breath, I'd pause to notice what was happening and when. I was often holding my breath when I was doing something stressful, and I was always holding it when I was in a negative body image spiral. So now if I find myself holding my breath, I know to check in to see what else is going on so I can figure out how to address it.

As you get to know your body, breath, and feelings, patterns will continue to emerge.

Get Curious about Your Patterns

In addition to the breath pattern I just shared, another big pattern I noticed, which crept in when I was least expecting it, is how negatively I viewed my body—and myself by extension. I know you might be thinking, "Duh, how did she not know that?," but I didn't. Or, rather, I didn't know it was a pattern of thought that I could change. I thought it was an immutable, capital-T truth about my body and that what needed to change weren't my thoughts, but my body.

I've always had more than some reluctance to invoke the concept of body love, or loving your body. I mean, I do think it's a worthwhile thing to move toward (it's even part of the title of this book!). But, more often than not, I hear from people who think it sounds good—for everyone but them. That's why I prefer to talk more about the process and specifics than just tote the general concept. I find this helps because it's generally less easy for folks to resist, say, feeling your feet on the floor than loving your body, which can sometimes feel way too far out of reach. Because what I see is that when loving your body is put on the table first, it can be overwhelming. And it also connotes the idea that it's a destination, as though you'll arrive there on a day you'll clearly recognize and just brush your hands off and say to yourself, "Okay, that's done! What's next?"

But, of course, it's not like that at all.

It makes total sense to me that the idea of loving your body seems scary at best, impossible at worst. Many of us have a lifetime of experience receiving messages stating that, while other people's bodies may be okay to love, our own definitely isn't.

So because this pattern of thinking negatively about my body was so pervasive in my life, I want to spend a little time now with how I unwound one particular thread around that and how, once I began to tug at it, it led to loosening others.

The summer before I left for college, my mom and I were having one of those moments where you think you're just chatting, then suddenly the conversation gets deep. I vividly remember sitting on the black-and-white stool next to our trash can, on the side of the kitchen island. We started to talk about my impending move and what college life would be like. Then talk turned, as it often did, to my weight and how I needed to lose some. She stood to my left and looked at me with all sincerity and love and said, "Not everyone is like me. They won't love you as you are if you don't lose weight."

I don't remember many things people have said to me over the years in such clear detail, but that's one I can hear as though I'm still right there. Because for many, many years, I was.

These days (after many years of therapy!), I know what she meant. She meant that, in her experience of the world, how you look matters. And not just that: She also meant that society in general tends to punish bigger-bodied people, simultaneously making us think we're too much and also not enough. As we talked about earlier, my mom is hardly the originator of either of those ideas, and she's not wrong that fat bias exists. That's true in far too many ways and contexts in this world, and I know that she couldn't teach me another way that she herself hadn't learned. In that moment, though, I wasn't aware of any of that. I wasn't aware of anything at all except my own bodily signals of shame: the white-hot flash of heat, quick loss of hearing, and tunnel vision as everything dropped into a pit in my stomach.

Time stood still.

I don't remember what I said afterward. All I know is that though this wasn't a conscious decision, my longtime pattern of believing myself unlovable was cemented in that moment. I removed myself from the prospect of dating when she said that. I went off to college never expecting anyone to be interested in me (which wasn't hard to believe because it's not as if I'd elicited tons of interest in high school). I assumed I'd be single my whole life and never marry, so I set about doing what I enjoyed, not getting caught up in guy drama, as some of my friends did. I created an inner pattern of not expecting love, or really even like. So, eventually, when guys did express more overt interest in me, I was confused. I assumed they'd been set up on a dare by their friends, or that I was the butt of a joke. Or that they might be interested in private, but that they'd never deign to be seen with me in public.

So it should probably come as no surprise that, only six years later, when I found myself married, I didn't know how to receive or absorb my husband's love. Not really. I spent the next few years pushing it away, subtly and not so subtly, until I landed on the door of body acceptance. I was, at that point, decades into believing that my body was worthless, and that the same was true of me by extension. I also found myself imagining at every moment the affair my husband was surely deservedly having, or would be soon. It still surprises me to this day, though less so now, when he says he's happy and loves our life together. Some part of me that's stuck in that moment in my parents' kitchen still doesn't know why he stays, even though he never gives me any reason to think that. And I still have a near–panic attack anytime he wants me to go to a work function or have dinner with his friends, convinced as I am that they will look at him with pity when they see me and pull him aside and tell him that he could do better.

What I slowly came to realize is that though my husband's love did help me feel better about my body, it wasn't enough. I just thought, "Sure, he says he loves my body, but I somehow lucked onto the one person on earth who does, and I know it won't last. I wonder what's wrong with him?" I felt lucky, but like I was walking on quicksand. Because I found my own body so contemptible, I couldn't fully trust that he didn't, too.

Some part of me knew that this wasn't healthy thinking, so I mostly tried to keep those thoughts to myself. Though, of course, those things always have a way of coming out sideways, through making sure to always get dressed in a separate room or flinching from his touch when it landed on a body part I didn't like (which wasn't hard to find).

This was all happening around that time I'd tallied up the sixty-five diets I'd been on and realized I needed a drastically different approach to my health and caring for my body. So I started seeing a nutrition therapist who introduced me to books like *Intuitive Eating*,[1] which I'd encountered before but never explored. According to the authors, "Intuitive eating is an approach that teaches you how to create a healthy relationship with your food, mind and body—where you ultimately become the expert of your own body."[2] As I read that, an old cliché began to dawn on me: If you don't love yourself, no one else will, either.

Except, I actually think that's total BS. People very well may still love you if you don't love yourself. That was certainly true for me. What I find to be much truer, though, is that if you don't love yourself, it may be challenging to relax into the love of others, trusting that they're not just stringing you along until the moment they can leave you, no matter what the relationship is.

So I started to dip my toe into this idea of loving your body—and promptly made it a diet. Ha! Surprise, surprise, right? This showed up first as a food diet in the sense that my idea of intuitive eating was parceling out four baby carrots and declaring myself full. (What? That isn't what your body intuitively wants?) But it also showed up in only feeling worthy of my own love and affection if I ate those four carrots with glee, went around hungry, and didn't "give in" to the inevitable 3:00 p.m. hunger cravings.

I'd made my own love conditional on my ability to adhere to a diet, even though that was exactly what I was theoretically trying not to do.

It's no wonder, though, is it? From the perspective of hindsight, I see how that was really the only possible course for me for a while. I didn't have the skills, practice, examples, or self-trust to do anything else. The problem is that I didn't see it that way for years; rather, I saw it as yet another approach to taking care of myself that I'd failed.

Instead of deepening my self-trust, if anything, trying to love my body eroded it at first because I came it at from a very black-and-white, right-or-wrong place. I felt that if I couldn't get loving my body right, what could I get right?

What I eventually realized after several years of trying and "failing" at body love (mostly by going on more diets, feeling terrible, wishing for another way, then repeating that cycle over and over again) is that I was trying to start at what I imagined to be the finish line. Of course I couldn't start off loving my body, not with all the accumulated years of self-loathing I'd racked up.

I knew I needed to keep shifting the pattern of thinking I was unlovable, of relying on the newest diet rules vs. my body's signals, of falling back into the either/or way of relating to my body, and of assuming there's one right way (or one way at all) to love your body. Once I noticed the pattern, my next step was to look at what habits and routines I wanted to shift in order to write a new story about my life. After all, if you don't know where/how you're inscribing the pattern in the first place, it's challenging to know how to shift it.

Get Curious about the Everyday

One place I decided I had to start first was with what exactly happened when I got into a negative cycle about my body. One of the easiest places for me to notice this was with my then-frequent "closet fits," which is what I call those days when you feel like nothing you own looks good on you or fits. You know what I'm talking about, right? They're those days when all your clothes end up on the floor and you hate not only everything you own but yourself, too. Over time, I noticed this happened more on days when I was already stressed, and if I was stressed and feeling bad about my body for another reason? Game over.

The closet fits also told me something about the clothes themselves. When I tried to force my body into clothes that no longer fit well or that I just plain didn't like, I felt so much worse and fell quickly into the pit of body despair. Then, one day, this thought occurred to me: "What if I just get clothes that fit and that I like?"

Mind = blown.

I went to the store, determined not to worry about the size of the clothes I was buying. I can't say I was completely successful at that, but with keeping my focus on my comfort and not my size, I did manage to bring home a couple new pairs of pants and tops that fit and that I felt good in. It feels important to say here that I didn't get those clothes because I was suddenly totally happy with my body. Not even close! I did it by coaching myself—constantly—sometimes even out loud (though not in the dressing room). Anytime my thoughts derailed, I would tell myself: "You're here to find clothes that feel good. Do these pants work for that?" Similar to how yoga asked me to focus on one part of my body, thus bringing me out of the negative story I was constructing about my body, focusing myself on the task at hand over and over again while shopping allowed me to get home with the new clothes. And lo and behold if that didn't decrease the closet fits!

Sometimes the work we have to do to improve our relationship with our bodies is psychological and emotional. But other times, it's purely logistical. I think the closet fits made me feel bad about my body because they brought the confrontation front and center: My closet was a fantasy land full of clothes that had fit a previous iteration of my body, but my body was firmly in reality. And whenever there's a dissonance between fantasy and reality, there's often a sense of things not fitting together the way you want—in this case, literally.

So once I realized I might be able to feel better just by getting a few new articles of clothing, I felt an enormous sense of relief. Not happiness necessarily; at that time, that would have required me to wake up with a new, thin body. But I was so sick of the daily struggle that relief felt like a very close second. And even though I still really wanted that body at the time, I comforted myself with the thought that these new clothes would at least make me feel better for now while I waited on that magical body to arrive.

Once I got the new clothes, I was able to give a little more attention to the stress/closet fit pattern. If I followed the logic of the closet-fit situation, I would have thought: "Oh, I just need to never feel stress again! That will help!" And, of course, I'm sure that would help. But considering that I wouldn't be human in that scenario, I'm not sure how well it would work.

So what I did instead is become more observant of the pattern. When I was stressed about work or people in my life, I started telling myself before getting dressed in the morning that it might feel harder than usual, but that's okay. That it wasn't about my body, but just that everything was harder than usual right now.

Yep, I gave myself another little pep talk before even opening the closet doors!

And you know what? It helped! Acknowledging that a closet fit might happen due to a predictable response to stress seemed to take the steam out of it. And over time, I added to my mini pep talk by encouraging myself to choose something easy, that I knew fit well, and that I was comfortable in. Sometimes I'd even pick it out the night before if things in my life were really hard. No drama.

This is why I prefer to talk about moving toward being body-affirming as opposed to body-loving or even body-positive. Because the closet fits weren't resolved by loving myself more, at least not in the sense of rubbing my arm and lovingly telling myself that I'm beautiful exactly as I am, which is what I always thought it meant. Instead, it came from practical, body-affirming details and observation of my natural patterns and everyday habits, born out of curiosity.

Now, one could certainly argue that doing those things is being loving to your body or being body-positive. I wouldn't disagree with that. But it's not usually what's folks think of when they hear "body-loving" or "body-positive," which tend to evoke bubble baths, endless cheer, and beatific smiles. I've had thousands of conversations over the years with people who are interested in body acceptance and say things like this: "But I don't *feel* positive about my body." Then I'd have to explain how being body-positive doesn't mean *feeling* positive toward your body at all times. Same with body love: It doesn't mean you never feel anything less than loving toward your body, but more that you're cultivating a loving relationship with your body.

The same could certainly be said of "body-affirming" and "body-accepting," except that those two seem to be at least slightly less loaded terms for most people. None of these terms imply they're something you do at all times, no matter what, or that with one little "slipup," you're out. But way too many of us think this way—myself definitely included. I can't even possibly begin to count how many times I thought I'd "failed" at body acceptance! "Well, I gave that a go, but I just spent the last three hours feeling like crap about my body, so I guess the jig is up."

No, no, no, no, no.

Of course I still have times where I don't feel good about my body. I spent many, many years cultivating that pattern! It makes sense that I can't throw it out, especially entirely, in a small amount of time. If a similar time line is true for you, I want you to hear me here: Body acceptance isn't a diet, where I'm promising you overnight success—or, on the generous side, two weeks to a new you. I'm telling you right now that it's going to take time. The difference is that the time you're spending in this practice is further deepening, not eroding, your self- and body-trust.

Get Curious about the Bigger Picture

So this is where you start, which is where I did, too: curiosity and feeling what's happening right here, right now. After I got married and started my body acceptance journey, I was able to see how that one conversation with my mom had taken how I already felt about my body—bad—and solidified it into something so immovable that it just seemed like the cold, hard truth. But once I noticed that pattern of thinking I was unlovable, I got to see and unwind it from my life and my relationships. That resulted in noticing how I responded to my husband out of default patterns that had nothing to do with him, the slow undoing of my need to be on a diet, and the closet fits, among many others.

None of this could have happened without first simply noticing what was going on in my body. And that's not because doing so gave me a flashback or a flash of insight and I could suddenly see all my patterns clearly. Rather, it's because awareness has to start somewhere, and being on my yoga mat on a regular basis, being asked to tune in again and again to awareness, gave me the space to become more comfortable with the process and practice until it just felt like how I operate in the world.

And as curiosity about my patterns continued to grow along with my self-awareness and body awareness, I realized I had more beliefs I needed to challenge in order to move forward.

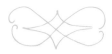

PRACTICES

Getting Curious on the Yoga Mat

A great place to begin getting curious about what's going on with your body is on your yoga mat. One way to do that is by asking yourself questions. Why questions? Because they open a space for possibility and curiosity, and that's a space that's ripe for exploration and deepening your practice. Some examples while on the yoga mat include:

* What's happening with my foot (or any body part, perhaps one that is sometimes harder for you to notice or one that's a focal point of the pose)?

* How am I breathing here?

* What could I do to make myself even 10 percent more comfortable?

* What can I stabilize, elongate, or strengthen (depending on what's relevant to the pose)?

* Where can I relax?

* What story am I telling myself about my body right now? Or about this pose?

✳ What does my body need in this moment? How can I meet that need?

✳ What does my body want in this moment? How can I meet that want?

You may find as you try out these different questions that you want to stick with one for a while. That can be so powerful because you get to see how your response shifts over time. You may also find your own questions that resonate for you (I hope you will!).

A word if you ask a question and don't get an answer, or get criticism from your inner critic instead: First, you are *so* not alone. This is like the start of any new conversation—sometimes a bit bumpy with lots of awkward silences. Don't let that deter you; you're just getting into your groove, which takes times. So if you don't get an answer, simply shrug your shoulders and move on. All you do is keep asking; when your body is ready, it will answer. If you get a negative answer from your inner critic, apply what we'll be talking about in the next chapter, which is how to challenge voices like that.

Get Curious Off the Yoga Mat

You can definitely engage in the process of getting curious when off your yoga mat, too! Similar to what we talked about with being present, you could answer some of the questions above at natural transition points in your day. For example, you might ask yourself what you need as you start your day, or what you want as you move from afternoon into evening.

Another way getting curious works off your mat is when you happen to notice something about your body or feelings. For example, let's say you're going about your day when all of the sudden you find yourself criticizing your body. That is the perfect time to stop and get curious! You might ask yourself: "Oh, I'm being really negative. What's going on here?" Or "What has happened in my day so far before this critical voice rose up? Or what's coming up next?" As you stay curious about your responses (and again, you may not have any for a while), you may begin to notice some of your patterns, as we discussed earlier in this chapter.

Meditation: Mind Observation

In addition to having a way to get curious about your body, it's useful to have a way to check in with your mind. I think of yoga *asanas*, or the poses, as the doorway into observing the body. By practicing the poses with attention and kindness, we learn to notice what's happening in the body—what it needs and what it doesn't need. And while this process certainly engages the mind, it doesn't always have the same level of awareness of the mind's patterns because it's focused on the body's patterns.

What's wonderful about meditation is that it does for the mind what yoga does for the body—it helps you observe your own patterns. Because it's not until you notice, for example, how and when your mind falls down a hole and you feel negatively about your body that you can start to shift it.

It's important to note that meditation is not about stopping thinking entirely. That's a common misconception. Rather, meditation is inner observation and awareness. One of the techniques I like most for meditation is a simple (though, again, not necessarily easy) observation of the breath. Here's how you can try it:

* Begin while you're seated in a comfortable position—on the floor, in a bed, whatever is available to you. Lengthen your spine as much as possible. You can also lie down if sitting isn't possible for you.

* Once in position, breathe at your regular pace.

* After several breaths like that, continue at your own pace while you begin to direct your attention to the breath. You can do this several ways: by feeling the breath entering in and exiting out your nostrils; by noting the rise and fall of your chest (maybe even placing one hand on your heart to make the connection clearer); or by observing the rise and fall of your belly (you could also place one hand on your belly if you're doing this one). Another option either in addition to or instead of the others, is to count your breath: inhaling to a count of 1; exhaling to a count of 2. You continue that process until you get to 10, and then you start back at 1 again.

* Any time your attention wanders from your breath (which may be at 10 or, if you're like me, 1½), gently bring it back. The

moment of noticing your attention has wandered is pure gold! That is very far from a sign of failure. It's actually a complete success—*because you noticed*. The whole point is noticing, so whenever you notice that your attention has drifted, celebrate another opportunity to bring it back.

 Continue this process for however long you'd like, but keep it simple. Two minutes a day is better than thirty minutes one day a month because consistency is what allows you to observe your own reactions and patterns.

As you continue your meditation process, you'll begin to observe your default mental escapes from paying attention. Some of mine (because I have many!) include thinking that I'm bored, that meditation is pointless, or that I don't have time for it; fidgeting constantly; worrying about anything and everything; obsessing about a weird feeling I just had and how it must be the sign of an undiagnosed terminal illness; replaying conversations from the past or imagining future conversations; listing all the things I don't like about my body; and on and on, ad nauseam.

This all matters to body acceptance because, guess what? How you hide and escape from yourself in meditation likely also has some major resonance for how you do the same with your body. After all, does thinking that body acceptance is boring, pointless, or sure to lead to a terrible outcome sound familiar? I'm guessing it does. For me, I know it does. But the more I see those patterns, the easier it becomes for me to break the negative body cycle I'm in.

For example, one of my patterns is quitting. If I don't like something (like meditation, but also anything in life), my first instinct is to say it's not for me and quit. I'm not a fan of the sticking-it-out strategy, at least not by default. As I saw myself do this time and again with meditation, though, I became more aware of it in my everyday life. Hard event coming up that I'm nervous about? Why not cancel it?! Tough conversation I need to have with a friend? Never mind! Continue the everyday, often tedious and boring process of body acceptance? No thanks!

Now when I notice a desire to quit or cancel something, I know it's a red flag. This isn't to say it's never appropriate for me to quit or cancel; sometimes it absolutely is—if I've overcommitted, said yes just to be nice but never really wanted to, am doing something that isn't a good idea for me or isn't working, and the like. But other times, wanting to quit is masking what's really true: that what I'm doing scares me on some level and that I don't enjoy feeling that level of vulnerability, so rather than doing it, I'd prefer to do nothing.

Quitting may not even be close to your pattern. But the beautiful thing about meditation is that it can show you what is. And it's from that place of knowing yourself, your reactions, patterns, and habits that you can see body acceptance as the path that it is and know that every detour is just that—not a fall completely off the map.

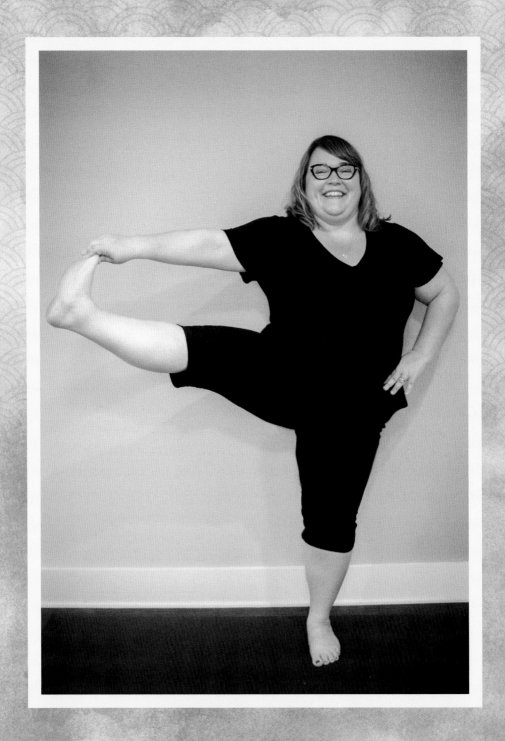

Challenge What You Know.

(Yes, I Mean Everything.)

As you get curious and come to know the current truth of yourself and your body through your felt experience, you will inevitably run into some beliefs you've been carrying around (for goodness knows how long!) that you can finally challenge to see what's still true for you.

Because when it comes to our bodies, *so much* of what we think about them isn't informed by our body's actual experience at all, but rather by others' expectations and opinions of them (which are, of course, also informed by yet others' expectations and opinions).

Breaking free of this cycle, while challenging, is also one of the most liberating things you can do for yourself. Because as you do this more and more, other people and societal expectations no longer define your worth or what's best for you: You do.

Which brings us to the first major thing we need to challenge: language— who gets to define us and how we define ourselves.

Challenge What You Know about Naming Your Body

Recently on social media, someone commented on one of my photos: "I don't think curvy means what you think it does."

Eye roll. Hard.

Probably thinking he's the first person to tell me I'm fat and not curvy, this person phrased his comment in the form of a wake-up call, as though he were doing me a favor. "Thank goodness for this random dude," I thought. "I've been getting it wrong all along!"

Except: not.

Because if there's one thing I've learned from talking, writing, and teaching about bodies of all shapes and sizes, it's this: There are no universally loved or uniformly used words to describe bodies.

So here's the thing: I do use the term fat to describe my body. However, I get more negative pushback when I *do* use it, not when I *don't*.

When I use the term fat to describe my body, I hear lots of "You're not fat! You're beautiful!" and other variations on that theme.

While I appreciate people trying to give me a compliment, they kind of make my point for me. I'm fat *and* beautiful. The two are not mutually exclusive, even though our culture certainly tries to convince us that they are.

People often ask me how I came up with the name Curvy Yoga. And, honestly, it was just one of those things. I was thinking of possibilities, and when it popped in my mind, I knew it was right.

Curvy resonates with me and with the many other people who tell me they connect with it because I find it to be both clear and friendly/welcoming. When I was very new on my body acceptance journey, I found it incredibly difficult to name or label my body in any way. No word described how I wanted my body to be, even though many might have described how it actually was.

I wasn't yet ready to own my body at all—not as curvy, much less as fat. So I chose curvy because I believe it invites people in who otherwise might be hesitant to even dip their toe near the water of body acceptance, much less in it, no matter what the actual shape/size of their body.

Of course, that doesn't mean it's universally loved. Like any term to describe a body, some people like it and other people don't. The objections range from too cute to too euphemistic to too gendered to not political enough to not accurate. The only objection I've ever heard that I didn't see coming was when someone said she almost didn't come to a class I was teaching because she thought "curvy" meant that we'd be moving our bodies in curving shapes à la Cirque du Soleil.

These days, I feel very comfortable calling myself and my body curvy, large, round, big, and, yes, fat. But those have all been a long time coming, especially the last one.

Like I mentioned, I'm okay with calling my own body fat. I believe deeply in reclaiming this word as a neutral descriptor, just like short or tall. I also understand, though, why people rebuff it as a word to describe their body—because other people use it as a weapon. This tiny three-letter word is loaded with cultural baggage. The connotations of fat these days encompass lazy, dirty, morally bankrupt, unhealthy, irresponsible, yet also somehow responsible for our national debt and the downfall of society: pretty much all the "bad" things you can say about someone. Did you know body tissue had this much power? Me, neither.

Naming your own body in safety is something that has been taken from many of us. Whether through trauma, medical expectations, judgments from loved ones, bullying as children (and adults), disordered eating, illness, injury, or any other number of things that happen to our bodies over the course of a lifetime, many of our bodies have been subject to others' labels and definitions.

Taking back the right to name your own body is a key step on the path to body acceptance. It's a moment of stepping into your own power and saying,

"This is my *curvy, differently abled, older, gorgeous, fat, slim, survivor* body."

Because once you make that kind of proclamation, adding a follow-up of "And I love it" isn't too far behind.

So that's why I intend to keep calling myself curvy. And large, beautiful, fat, short, round, lovely, big, and whatever else I want, whenever it feels appropriate for me.

And that's also why I intend to keep making space for others to do the same. I will never insist on people using any particular label (or not) because that doesn't support my vision of body acceptance or how yoga calls you into it. In yoga, you connect with your inner wisdom and move from that place. And you'd better believe your inner wisdom will have something to say about what feels safe and okay for you to call your body at any given moment.

Also, as with everything in life, how you describe your body may change over time. That has certainly been true for me. And the same is true for another area where challenging beliefs is absolutely instrumental: food.

Challenge What You Know about Food

I mentioned earlier that I tried my hand at Intuitive Eating, but I didn't tell you the best part yet: how I found it. You've done desperate middle-of-the-night Internet searching, right? That's usually the worst idea possible, but in one of my dark nights of the Internet, I happened upon Intuitive Eating. Although I had *no* clue what it meant at the time, I liked the idea of it. My understanding then was that you learned how to "trust" (and yes, scare quotes are required because that's how made-up I thought this idea was at the time) your body to tell you what and how much to eat. "A diet I make up myself," I thought. "How great!"

I knew I'd need some assistance to make this plan work, so I was fortunate to find that nutrition therapist I mentioned earlier. (Later in the process I also worked with a psychotherapist for help with this and related issues. I can't recommend therapy highly enough!) This wonderful woman coached me through months of beginning the painful process of reconnecting with my hunger. She also introduced me to Health at Every Size® (HAES), which is an approach to health that focuses on healthy behavior, not weight loss. Though I'd long suspected something was broken in me and I could never feel full, it turned out that something quite different was at play. What I found instead is that I had no clue when I was hungry or when I was full, unless I was all the way to a 10 on the hunger scale, so stuffed they called it Thanksgiving-full.

It turns out that sixty-five different diets over twenty-plus years had caused me to completely disconnect from my own body's cues. I wasn't broken at all, but I was so numb from relying on external diet rules and outside advice that I'd lost my ability to listen to my internal advice. So every day, every time I ate, I charted my hunger and satiety on a scale from 1 (so hungry you'd eat the next thing that crossed your path) to 10 (unbutton your pants and take a nap). I'd mark how hungry I was before I ate, and how full I was afterwards.

For most of the time that I engaged in that process, I lied about my answers: a 3 before and a 7 afterwards. I didn't lie because I didn't want to tell the truth, but because I didn't know the truth and I was too ashamed to admit it. I was ashamed because it felt like something I should be able to do, and when I couldn't, it felt like yet another failure in the body realm for me. First, I couldn't get diets "right," and now I couldn't even get hunger "right?!" I was extremely frustrated with myself because I was used to being competent in most areas of my life, and in this I had to be a brand-new beginner. Like a pretraining-wheels beginner. So I went with what seemed like safe and reasonable guesses, varying it up a little from time to time so as not to be too obvious. I wasn't even entirely convinced that *anyone* could do more than take a shot in the dark, though my nutritionist assured me people could.

As I continued to work with my nutrition therapist, on a gut level I felt so relieved by what she was teaching me.

But it was also scary as hell.

After a couple of heady months spent loosening my diet rules and not hopping on the scale, I freaked out when one day I hopped on and found I'd gained ten pounds (4.5 kg). Clearly, this trusting your body nonsense was only *really* applicable to thin people who could afford to do it.

So for the next year, I got back on the diet train straight to hate-yourself town. But when another year of failed experiments left me at the same weight as when I'd started, I knew that my nutrition therapist had been right all along. The problem wasn't me; the problem was how the diets disconnected me from my innate wisdom.

This process was tricky for me because I was learning to navigate my way between a diet and an approach to eating. To me, a diet imposes external guidelines on what I eat—whether or not that makes sense for my body, whether or not it's sustainable—and it's solely focused on weight loss. Some examples of this are obvious: You might remember the cabbage soup diet from years ago. Pretty much all you do is eat cabbage soup. It's easy to see how your body would not get what it needs over the short term (not to mention the long term!) from just eating cabbage and broth.

The less obvious diets are the ones we see that are ostensibly about "health" but are really just some variation of the cabbage soup diet in disguise. So today that might look like a "cleanse," which is said to be about health (with weight loss as a welcome side effect) but which research has thoroughly debunked.[1]

It took me a long time to challenge what I know about food, health, and eating, to begin to discern what it truly means for me to eat intuitively. What helps me navigate those tricky gray areas now is challenging a few things. If I find something that's only a list of a million rules and the consequences of breaking those rules are imminent death and the destruction of the planet, then I know I've run into something more like a diet in its rigidity. Yet another thing I watch for (and this is the biggie) is the focus. I find that the focus of a diet is almost exclusively on weight loss (whether this is explicit or implicit, because diet gurus have noticed that we're onto them a bit these days and have sometimes changed their language more to "health" or "lifestyle change" in response), whereas the focus of a way of eating is nourishing yourself how you uniquely need to be and feeling good—whatever helps you boost your energy, sleep well, get the nourishment you need, move your body, and so on. Ultimately, a way of eating is something that grows out of a long and ongoing conversation with your body, not yet another arbitrary diet plan (of course, if you do have specific food allergies or needs, you can find a body positive–health provider to help you navigate). One of the biggest challenges in making this switch is that you have to also challenge what you know about health.

Challenge What You Know about Health

I started blogging a year or so after I started teaching yoga. And about a year into blogging, my writing started to receive a small amount of attention. And, of course, when you attract any modicum of attention on the Internet, you open yourself to responses from folks who don't agree with you.

In general these days, I don't read anything written about me, and I *definitely* never read the comments section online. I mean, I don't have whole days to give myself over to the inevitable shame I will feel when I get sucked into reading negative comments. So I just don't do it.

But that first year in, I was earnest and felt I somehow owed it to—well, I don't know to whom. But I thought I should read these things, so I did. Mostly I could just write them off as people who didn't get where I was coming from, or who disagreed with me, neither of which I see as about me.

That is, until I read one written by a former yoga teacher of mine.

I don't remember the exact details of the post, but I do recall the gist was something like this: "This idiot says it's okay to be fat. Health at Every Size was invented as a justification for fat people. It is not okay to be fat, and anyone who thinks so—especially Anna Guest-Jelley of 'Curvy' Yoga—is a moron."

I felt the familiar flush of shame flood from my head to my toes as I read my former teacher's post about how much my existence and viewpoint offended him. But I also felt somewhat weirdly amused because I could tell he didn't remember I'd ever been in class with him.

In that moment, I felt free. This wasn't written by some scary person, but by a bookish yoga teacher who I knew to be completely unintimidating. I didn't think that justified his harsh characterizations of me, but he did prove to me why this work of challenging what we know about weight, health, and bodies for people of every shape and size matters.

When I first heard about Health at Every Size,[2] I couldn't believe it. And I don't mean that I thought it was awesome. I mean, I literally could not believe it was possible.

As Dr. Linda Bacon says in her book *Health at Every Size: The Surprising Truth About Your Weight*, "When you stop trying to control your weight through willpower, your body starts doing the job for you—naturally, and much more effectively."[3] It does not mean, as is incorrectly assumed by many, that every person is healthy at every size. Rather, it works to break the weight/health connection by reminding us that seeing a person's body and/or knowing her weight doesn't tell us anything but what her body looks like or what her weight is. Because just as there are unhealthy thin people (of course! I'm sure you know some!), there are healthy fat people, and vice versa. When you think about it this way, I think many of us realize what a no brainer it is. Because of course something as complex as health can't be boiled down to only one factor.

People's health is based on many different factors—genetics, environment, past history, eating/movement habits, and so on. So to think that one thing—weight—can tell you everything you need to know about your own health, much less another person's is silly. But as a society, we love oversimplification and stereotyping because it gives us an "easy" way to communicate. Yet as is always the case with stereotyping, we lose the humanity of the individual, which can never be captured with such broad strokes.

And for those of you who are reading this and thinking something like "But wait, this isn't just stereotyping! Being fat *is* bad!," I get it. Most of us have been taught to believe this. But studies continue to prove that wrong, despite the persistence of the myth in mainstream society.[4] You can find many of those studies in Dr. Bacon's book, among other places.

Weight, like health, is individual.[5] But it's easier to make sweeping assumptions that the only thing going on with a fat person's health is his weight than to look into what else might be happening. There are many stories of people not getting the health care they need, and even dying, because their health-care professional wouldn't look past their weight.[6] This has even happened to me!

After a fall and a not-clear x-ray, I was told my ankle was sprained, to rest it, and to come back if it wasn't feeling better in a few weeks, despite my protestations that I could feel the broken bone. So in a few weeks I went back because not only was it not better, it was even more painful than before. My doctor proceeded to tell me how I probably still felt bad due to my weight. She then proceeded to tell me I should try a weight loss program (which, as you know, I had—dozens of times by this point) and all about how her husband had lost a bunch of weight on one particular weight loss program recently. When I pressed her, she finally said I could go see an orthopedist "if I wanted," though it was clear she thought it was pointless. I said that I did, went to see him a few days later, had a more in-depth scan done, and lo and behold—my ankle had been broken the whole time. The only problem? It was now too late to put it in a cast. As a result, my ankle still gives me pain sometimes more than a decade later, and it has negatively affected my gait and posture because it never healed properly.

All this happened because my doctor (who wasn't my doctor after that!), assumed the only reason a fat person would continue to be in pain was because of her weight. But would she have assumed the same about a thin person? I highly doubt it.

I think more of us than we think know that focusing on losing weight doesn't work, particularly in the long term. We know because we or someone we know (usually multiple someones) are living examples of the experiments we've been running on ourselves in this regard. And we've already talked about the many reasons we're led to believe the old "it's not you, it's me" thing that diets make us feel toward ourselves.

With an approach like Health at Every Size, you're free to live what I think many of us already know, at least on a gut level—that shifting your focus to caring for yourself now regardless of your weight will lead to a much happier life and even a healthier one as you get your body out of the starvation cycle of diets.

As we move toward a more peaceful relationship with our body's health, we can do the same thing with our mind—by looking at how we talk about our bodies, both with others and ourselves.

Challenge What You Know about Self-Talk

I can't remember when it started, but I'd definitely say that elementary school is not an exaggeration. That's at least when I have a conscious memory of it. I remember talking with one of my friends on the last day of probably fourth grade about how we were the biggest girls in class. We whispered together during a dark gym assembly, me reassuring my friend her body was okay because, hey, look how much worse mine was and her doing the same for me. I remember the sense of relief I felt talking with her. At that time, "biggest" meant "tallest" as well as "heaviest." Shortly after that, though, I stopped getting taller.

This is just an early example of one of the primary ways that I have bonded with women in my life—through mutual self-loathing and talking badly about our bodies. I can remember so many different occasions where this came up—all through school, in church camp bathrooms, college dorms, cars on the way out for the night, and on and on. I remember the pockets of anxiety waiting for a night to begin and filling that time with the fidgety beautifying so many women engage in—last-minute lipstick swipes, hair changes, shoe swaps. It's like the only way we learned to affirm each other is by not only commiserating but one-upping in the ugly/fat/terrible clothes department. I have so often shown "love" to my friends by answering their question of "Tell me the truth: Do I look fat in this?" with "No way! And I don't know why you're even saying that. You look so great; just look at how gross I look in this dress!"

Over time, this really started to grate on me. It also started to become more and more conspicuous as I continued gaining weight and I could no longer even shop at the same stores with my friends.

So several years ago, I decided to give all this a break and try not putting my body down for a week. I was in for a week of no comments about how big my butt looked, no "comforting" a friend by telling her how much worse I looked compared to her, no bemoaning how much I'd regret eating that brownie later. I did this to cultivate some awareness in my life. And that's what I told people when they asked about it—"Oh, I'm just trying this out as an interesting social experiment to deconstruct the ways that women talk about their bodies." I figured if I made it sound academic, people would leave me alone and not ask me the real reason I was doing it.

The real reason I stopped engaging in this kind of conversation was that I didn't know what else to do. I could see that I was about to get stuck in it for the rest of my life (or, if you take away the melodrama, at least for the foreseeable future), and since that had already been my reality for close to thirty years, I knew I needed to do something to shake things up.

Though it was challenging, that week became a turning point for me. Releasing myself from the pressure of talking badly about myself out loud also gave me just the smallest bit of inner relief. I'm not going to exaggerate this story and say that after a week I never talked badly about my body again, though; that's just not true.

However, what is true is that through that tiny crack, I started to see how my life could be different. What I found is that by limiting myself from talking badly about my body to others, I let my foot off the gas of a similar (though usually much harsher) inner narrative. By refraining from talking badly about my body both externally and internally, even in the smallest ways, I found new ways to figure out what my unique body needed and to connect—with both myself and others.

You might consider a similar experiment yourself. There's something about bringing that kind of talk into your consciousness that lets you see just how pervasive it is. You can do the same with your self-talk. For example, you could try a one-week experiment where you keep a tally of any time you catch yourself putting your body down. Doing this helped me notice the recurring themes in my self-talk, as well as notice just how often it was happening. When I noticed the recurring themes, it became more possible for me to question and dismiss them: "Oh, this again. What a broken record." I'd also tell myself things like "Wow, this one is persistent!" Doing that helped me roll my eyes when those thoughts crept back in rather than actually believe them. The same is true for me now—though I definitely notice how much less often my self-talk is as negative as it once was, an occasional thought will pop back up, and when it does, I shake my head and move on. Those thoughts don't have the power to ruin my day anymore.

And neither do the thoughts I once had about who gets to practice yoga and who doesn't.

Challenge What You Know about Yoga

Health at Every Size informs Curvy Yoga not only because of the soundness of seeing health as individual, but also because of how it connects with yoga philosophy. Like HAES, yoga is a practice for turning inward and getting to know yourself.

The inner listening that yoga facilitates and encourages keeps me coming back to the mat and allows anyone in any body to participate in the practice. Because as you get to know your body and how to adapt the poses to it, your ability to listen within grows deeper.

Like many things in life, yoga poses are often taught (even to teachers in training) on an assumed thin, fit, able-bodied, and fairly flexible body. In some ways, that makes learning and teaching the poses as a teacher easier. In that context, there is a "right" and "wrong" way to do a pose, and your job as a teacher is to help students get their body to move into the "right" way.

The only problem? Way more of us are not already thin, fit, able-bodied, and flexible than are. Even if you're one, two, or three of those, very few folks are all four. So that means the vast majority of students will not be able to do the "right" version of the pose. And that tends to encourage one of two things for many people: (1) dropping out (or not starting in the first place) or (2) forcing your body into a version of a pose that isn't right for you.

Of course, learning to do new things isn't wrong, nor is challenging yourself. And it makes sense that people cannot come to yoga, no matter their body shape/size/ability, and do every pose right out of the gate. But too often what happens is that people do whatever they can to force their body into the look of a pose and compromise their alignment, balance, and safety in the process because they're not given pose options that actually work for them.

The other thing that happens is that people get discouraged or drop out because they feel like they'll only be able to participate if they get a new body. So here's the good news: You don't need a new body to start yoga. Which is great, because guess what? You're not getting one.

But don't worry, because neither is anyone else.

The idea of a "new body" is a myth we're sold. Plain and simple. It could never be anything but that because we all logically know we're never getting a new body—that even if our body changes in any way (which, of course, it does constantly), it's not new.

Losing weight doesn't make your body new. Neither does gaining weight. Neither does gaining muscle. Or suffering an injury. Or having an illness. Or dying your hair. Or having plastic surgery. Or having a baby. Or breaking a bone.

Some of these things may make your body feel different, but feeling, looking, or even functioning differently does not a new body make.

We're all still us, which is better than it may sound. Because the other side of this "new body" myth is that it presupposes that new = better. Not only does this insult your "old" body, it also implies that all change is for the better, so that when something changes about our bodies that we don't like, we're doubly hard on ourselves.

But here's the truth—for you, me, and everyone else—no matter what your body's shape, size, age, or ability is, it's yours. And that means it's with you for the long haul—an ever-present reminder that the only true possibility if we want even a modicum of inner peace and freedom is to learn how to accept and love the one body we have.

Because even though it will change in various ways over time, nothing and no one is with us more than our one, only-new-on-day-one body. It shows up more for us than anyone or anything ever will, even when we're not happy with it, even when we wish it were different, even when we lambaste it.

So you can just take that off the table: You don't need to become more flexible, thinner, "more in shape" (whatever that means), or anything else to try yoga. You just have to show up.

Of course, that's sometimes easier said than done.

I've had mini panic attacks in my car in the parking lots of more than one yoga studio and turned around and gone home. I've also gotten halfway there, freaked, and steered my car to the mall instead.

Sometimes all the good intentions in the world couldn't outweigh the nerves that arose when I contemplated going to a new yoga class as a fat person. Even to this day, when I know I can find a version of any pose that will work for me, no matter what the teacher offers (or doesn't), I can still feel my nervous system clanging around, asking me: Is this *really* a good idea?

Trying anything new can be anxiety-producing. I totally get that's not a size-specific thing. But when something like yoga is portrayed in the mainstream as the domain of the already thin, fit, and über-flexible, and you're not those things, it only makes sense that you might feel an extra layer of fear. That's how our culture works: On the whole, it says who's in—and who's not.

This is also how any form of oppression works in our society: Those whom society has decided to favor (read: white, thin, fit, able-bodied, male, heterosexual, middle-class-at-minimum) move through the world with greater ease than the rest of us. On the whole, the rest of us are made to feel we're not measuring up in some way when we don't fit those criteria, though they're arbitrary criteria that Western society decided to privilege in the first place. So that's what privilege means: Some people move through our world with more ease due to certain traits society deems "better."

For example, one form of privilege is thin privilege. People who live in thin bodies are generally held up as beautiful, desirable, and the ideal we should all be working toward. Except, of course, all bodies are different, and every body can't be a thin body, for a host of different reasons.

So what happens when thin privilege shows up in yoga, as it often does? A self-perpetuating cycle is created. Yoga is taught to thin students, who feel good about participating because it's geared to their body, so then they become thin teachers who have likely only been taught to teach thin students, who teach thin students who become thin teachers and so on and so on. Soon, you're to the point where when you ask any random people on the street who yoga is for, they're more likely than not going to identify a thin, fit, über-flexible, able-bodied person.

All this to say that when fat people go to yoga classes, it's with less privilege than thin people. This has nothing to do with individuals, who may or may not "feel" that they have more or less privilege, but rather with our society as a whole. For example, a thin person may say she's not privileged because she grew up poor. But that's not accurate. Because while that means she doesn't have as much *class* privilege as someone who did not grow up poor, she still has thin privilege. One form doesn't negate another. We almost all have areas where we have privilege and others where we don't.

For example, as a fat woman, I don't have thin privilege. But as someone who is white, heterosexual, cisgendered, with advanced degrees, and who grew up middle class, I have an abundance of privilege in those areas. It's not either/or.

When we know that, generally, thin privilege rules the day in yoga classes (though, thankfully, that is slowly starting to shift), it makes sense that going to class as a curvy person can be a big deal that is intensified even more at the intersections of other identities. It also makes sense that even when you become more comfortable with your body, there still may be different contexts that bring it up again.

Some people don't think that this is an issue, though, or rather they don't think it should be. The most common complaint I hear people have about Curvy Yoga is that some folks don't think it's needed because they think all students should be able to practice in all classes comfortably. These people fear that classes that are explicitly welcoming to curvy bodies are stigmatizing and silo students into never being able to participate anywhere else. But, of course, nothing could be further from the truth. Curvy classes aren't the *only* place to practice; they're just *a* place to practice for people who want it. These classes are no different than classes for seniors, pregnant women, people with back pain or any other type of specialized class. People have come together in solidarity and community when they so choose to get the support they want in a way that works for them, whether yoga related or not, for probably as long as we humans have been around. And even if all classes became curvy friendly overnight, I still think there'd be a place for Curvy Yoga classes because of the intentional community they create.

The next thing people share with me is usually something along the lines that yoga doesn't care what you look like. Here's what I always tell those folks: I agree! It would be wonderful if all yoga classes were accommodating of all bodies! But we don't yet live in that world. Because while the practice of yoga doesn't care what you look like, much of the culture certainly does, and yoga teachers, classes, studios, and students are part of that culture.

The truth is that not every yoga class is designed to meet the needs of curvy bodies, not even classes called Beginners, Gentle, Hatha, or even

Restorative. Because many yoga teachers learn to teach students who live in thin, already flexible and able bodies, it's not the pace of the class that's most relevant, but the instructions and options that are included (or not).

Yoga instruction we see in most classes these days has come to us through a blend of yoga *asana*, gymnastics, aerobics, and more.[7] Like any other facet of culture, it is influenced and shaped by the current moment. This is why we see poses today that weren't around even twenty years ago, never mind more. With that in mind, it's even less surprising that current yoga instruction (and past yoga instruction) mostly targets the already thin—because all contemporary fitness culture (and society) does the same. And the types of yoga and fitness information that fat people typically receive, like "Try harder," "Go faster," "Sit this one out," or even "Use props" (if there's no information on *how* or *why* to use them) are nothing but shame-based so-called motivators, not truly relevant information about the needs of curvy bodies.

And these are just the technical, yoga pose–based reasons why creating space for curvy people to practice is important. The other reasons are based on the exclusion that many fat folks feel in yoga classes that do not offer, or sometimes even fail to attempt to offer, pose options that work for them, even in classes that are purportedly for everyone. Many of these classes do not offer more than one pose option, even if the teacher is well-intentioned in being welcoming (as many are). When yoga classes lack body diversity and relevant instruction, it's not difficult to realize that curvy folks may feel as if they're on the fringes—because they're often literally told to just hang out in Child's Pose (which is not even a comfortable pose as it's traditionally taught for many curvy-bodied people) while the rest of the class does the "real" poses (whether that message is conveyed implicitly or explicitly).

This isn't to say there aren't yoga teachers and classes that have raised their awareness about the thin privilege dynamic and consciously sought ways not only to *say* that their yoga is inclusive, but to enhance their skills in order to meet the needs of a variety of students. Blessedly, these teachers do exist, and their number is growing all the time.

I remember when I first started practicing yoga. The teachers gave the same instructions over and over again, and everyone else seemed to blissfully go along with them (though, in hindsight, I realize that probably wasn't even true). I, however, kept thinking: "*How* can I stand with my feet together here? My knees hurt!" or "Put my belly on my thighs?! It was there the second we leaned forward an inch (2.5 cm)!"

The underlying internal commentary I heard was simply this: "What's wrong with me?" "What's wrong with me?" "What's wrong with me?"

It's not a question I needed any time to answer, because I always knew the answer. I'd known the answer since I was a child: too fat, too fat, too fat.

When teachers don't acknowledge that more exists in their students' bodies than muscles and bones, they leave the rest to the imagination. And in a thin-privileged world, the "imagination" (because it's more like all the received messages up to that point) has a tendency to fill in the blank with this: "My body is wrong."

Because as we've discussed, whatever we keep in the silence is a ripe candidate for shame. And when teachers don't acknowledge that your belly may feel compressed in a forward bend and that you can simply step your feet a little wider or move it to make space, you're left to either stay and feel uncomfortable or, as is true for many people, assume that yoga isn't right for you and abandon the practice entirely.

This doesn't have to happen, though. With the necessary information to practice in a way that works for their bodies, curvy folks can then practice in any type or style of class they choose, including curvy-style classes or not. That's the beauty of all the yoga options available today: People can go with what works for them, not be forced to choose between struggle or not participating at all.

I've seen this so often as a teacher. When I first started Curvy Yoga, I assumed that the only people who would be into it would be other curvy folks like me. Boy, was I wrong.

From day one, I've had students of *every* shape and size in class. At first, I found myself thinking, "Have these thin folks gotten lost?" But soon, my mind and heart opened to just how many of us are affected by feelings of bodily disconnection and feelings of not measuring up, no matter what our body shape or size. I quickly realized through talking with my students that being in a body affirming space where everyone is given the support and tools they need to be in their own body and experience is a rare and powerful thing.

Here's the thing, though: Just because many shapes and sizes may attend curvy-type classes, that doesn't mean we can just get rid of the name, call the class "yoga for all" or something like that, and call it a day. Because I do think that drawing attention (and more importantly, knowledge) to the issue of curvy bodies in yoga classes is essential, as is letting folks know that these are places that are explicitly welcoming. Fat people do face unique stigma, bias, and discrimination based on their size that must be acknowledged and addressed. There truly are things that students and teachers need to know in order to help curvy students practice more comfortably. And as more of us bring this into our lives, practices, and communities, I think we're slowly moving away from a narrow (often literally) definition of yoga and into a more open and individualized practice that suits the needs of the user. This means considering the needs of curvy bodies as well as all others. We all benefit when the focus is on listening to our body within the parameters of safety because it gives all of us the permission to find what works for us. And it is from this place that the seed of body acceptance can grow.

Challenge What You Know about Body Image and Body Acceptance

When I was in my early twenties, I prided myself on being a feminist activist. I spent every day poring over the news, forwarding stories of injustices and online actions to friends. For me, that was a way into my feelings—I couldn't feel tears in my eyes about anything in my own life, but I could feel them spring up for the many harsh and unjust things in this world.

I cared about pretty much everything—except body image activism. Actually, that's even being too generous. I felt it was a complete waste of time. After people knew that digitally altering photos was a thing, I thought, what was left? Why would we waste our time with such petty nonsense when there was important work to do?

It wasn't until at least five years later that I realized why I balked at this work—it was mine, and I didn't want it. And it was mine in a way that I *really* didn't want. It wasn't just about media literacy, but about learning to be in my own body. And not only giving a lecture about it, but actually living it. It was about doing years of healing work—and always finding more just around the corner.

Yoga has an interesting relationship to body image. Though this is definitely starting to change due to the good work of many people, it has long been a practice that focuses on the body without considering how people feel *about* their body.[8] The mainstream representations of yoga we talked about earlier certainly haven't helped with this. Fortunately, more and more people are staking their own claim on representations of yoga by sharing images of their own bodies—all shapes, sizes, ages, genders, abilities, races, and more.

Something similar is now happening with body acceptance. For a long time it's been considered the domain of people who "need it," but now more and more of us are realizing what it can mean for our lives, no matter what our bodies look like or how they are perceived. Similar to what we talked about with yoga, though, it's easy for body acceptance to get co-opted—for companies to hop on board as a way to sell products or for people to even use it to sell cleanses, diets, or other "lifestyle changes." Putting a different face (or body) on these, though, doesn't change them. A diet is a diet, and if the representations of bodies have only changed from one woman who's a size zero to another one who's a size six, we can't declare that good enough. Because all that did was open the door half a centimeter wider, while still operating within almost the exact same paradigms of beauty and social acceptance as before, which still leaves most of us out in the cold.

Empowering media representations of diverse bodies can definitely inspire us on our body acceptance journey. When you see a fat body represented positively, it makes a little space in the collective consciousness. These images even encourage many people to get interested in body image activism or body acceptance in the first place.

But though we do need that work, that's not all we need. Because from there, we also have to look at what's next.

Body acceptance starts where you are and begins to move first not toward love but toward neutral. Because when you're in neutral, you're *in* your body. You're *embodied*, moving through the world, doing your thing. For most of my life, the daily stew I soaked in was negativity toward my body. But these days? It's not love or even positivity. It's neutrality. It's less feeling something *about* my body and more feeling something *in* my body.

What that means on a practical level is one thing we've already talked about: that my closet fits are much fewer and further between. It also means that I eat what I want when I want it (and no, it's not a pile of junk food at every waking moment, as many people fear when they begin trusting their body more around food). It's engaging in this practice we've been talking about—presence, get curious, challenge, and affirm.

Most days, I'm on the neutral/like end of the loathing/dislike/neutral/like/love continuum. I can tell the difference because on the dislike/neutral end, I start getting crabby. I also start berating myself: "Why did you eat that? Why haven't you done your yoga yet today? Get it together, Guest-Jelley!" (Yes, my inner voice actually says that!) When that drill sergeant voice cranks up, I know I'm about to tip over the ledge into the pit of loathing.

So when I see that coming, I do a little visualization. This came to me one day because I so often thought of that experience in the language I used above: on the ledge, about to fall into a pit. That's how it felt to me, that there was this teetering moment when I could go either way. So now when I feel that, I picture a tiny (as in pocket-sized) me on the ledge, teetering this way and that, about to fall into a dark, seemingly bottomless pit below. And then I see the current me pluck the tiny me up and set me far back from the ledge.

There's something about that moment: Knowing I can help myself, pulling myself far enough back that I can't possibly fall in, that resets my current moment. I remember with relief: Oh, right—I have a choice here. Falling into the pit is not inevitable. In fact, that was my mantra for quite some time: "Falling into the pit is not inevitable."

So if this is body neutral, what is body like or love? What I've found is that it's similar to any long-term loving relationship. When you're with someone on a regular basis (friend, parent, child, partner) and you love that person, most of your everyday experience is neutral/like. You're happy to be with her, but you're not actively feeling *love* for her at all times. You feel love actively when you make the time for it, or when you do something special together, or when you take a break from the day just to be together. During those moments, you remember: I am *so* lucky to get to love this person. She is just *wonderful*.

In my experience, the same is true of my relationship to my body. Most of the time, I do not actively feel love for it. This isn't because I don't love it, but rather because I don't think that active love is an inner state that we maintain at all times. Rather, it's something that infuses the everyday and comes into sharp focus at certain moments. So there are times now when I hear people at the table next to me in a restaurant putting their bodies down, and it surprises me because it's been years since I've done that, and I forget how grateful I am to be able to have other kinds of conversations with my friends. In moments like that, I feel filled with love toward my body and the relationship we've cultivated. Other times I feel love for my body clearly include when I'm out in nature and my body has just helped me take a hike. As we go along, I'm so filled up by nature and by getting to move through it that a feeling of love toward my body arises naturally.

Similar to relationships with other people, these moments of active love toward my body are just that—moments where I've stepped out of ordinary time to feel and appreciate the goodness around and within me. And also similar to relationships with others, there's an overall foundation of love that I've built over time, layered with trust, that allows love to permeate how I feel toward my body, even when it's not active and I'm not thinking, "Gosh, my body is so awesome!"

Because I think that's how most of us picture it at first, so far removed does it seem: that when we love our body, we'll be spending all our time skipping through fields, singing songs about body love, telling ourselves how awesome our bodies are. But, of course, that doesn't happen. Or maybe it happens for a short period of time, but it doesn't go on forever. What happens instead is you go about your day, not always thinking in the background about what this person or that person must be thinking about how terrible you look, or obsessing about what you ate or didn't eat, or feeling uncomfortable because you tried to stuff yourself into clothes that don't fit or don't feel good.

In other words, you become free to live your life with less commentary from the inner and outer peanut gallery of body negativity and with more absorption into whatever is in front of you moment to moment. You get to be an active participant in your life, not just wait around until some dreamed-of day in the future when your body is exactly how you want it to be and you can finally enjoy yourself.

Challenge What You Know about Showing Up

I want to reiterate what I said before about body acceptance being an active process. Too often, our society promotes the idea that if you accept your body, that means you're giving up on it. But I've found nothing to be further from the truth.

I think it's ridiculous that society has this idea that to accept your body means to throw in the towel and not care about yourself. I find that there's absolutely nothing passive about accepting your body. Because to truly accept your body means to be attuned to its ever-changing needs. You don't just figure out your body's needs one day and then—check!— mark that off the list.

Pretty much the opposite.

Accepting your body means being in conversation with your body. And as in any relationship, that only works when you're willing to listen on a deep and regular basis. To be responsive to changing needs. To try to meet a need one day only to find that, nope, that wasn't it, and try again. And it also means knowing that, of course, sometimes the conversation will be one-sided, or you won't talk for a while, and that doesn't mean the relationship is over or that either of you failed—just that it might be nice to pick back up again. This is not a relationship that's dependent on you or your body being, looking, feeling, or acting any way other than what's true in this moment.

I have never, ever, ever (I can go on, trust me) taken better care of my body than I do now, after years of working with body acceptance.

In my pre–body-accepting days, I didn't care about what my body was telling me, what my body needed, or anything but weight loss. That was the only thing I cared about *at all*. So if my diet consisted solely of carrots and broth, and I wasn't getting any nutrients, and I couldn't sleep, and I was the crankiest cranker who ever lived, I didn't care a whit. And goodness knows I truly couldn't care less about how I felt. I considered that a completely meaningless piece of information. I repeat: *All* I cared about was knocking the number on that scale down another tenth of a pound.

But these days? I do care about how I feel. Quite a bit. I care that I do movement I enjoy that gets my heart pumping sometimes because it feels good and is as much for my mental health as my physical health (lap swimming, hiking, and yoga!). I never even knew how much better I could feel mentally and emotionally when moving my body until body acceptance became part of my life, even in a tiny way, because up until then it had only been about discipline and "working off" times that "I was bad" and, you know, ate food. Was a human.

I also care about what I eat—that I eat a variety of foods that serve my needs in the moment. And that I don't throw myself into the gutter when I don't. I care that I don't eat things that give me migraines, drain my energy, or otherwise make me feel unwell. And that when I do eat something that doesn't make my body happy, I don't tell myself what a fraud and failure I am. I care that I don't become so obsessed with food that I can't enjoy a piece of cake at a friend's birthday party. I care that food can be what it is: nourishment, community, joy, and sustenance. And not what it isn't: an arbiter of whether or not I'm a good person.

I believe body acceptance is about discerning and supporting yourself in what health means for you on an intimate, daily level. It is weight-neutral, meaning that your weight just does what it does. Neither weight gain, nor weight loss, nor weight stability is demonized or lionized. Because weight isn't the point. Feeling as good as is currently possible, living *in* your body, nourishing yourself in the way that is appropriate for you, prioritizing whatever gives you mental and emotional freedom, is. Whatever your weight does from there is up to it. No matter what happens to your weight, it is never something that you have to apologize for, justify, or even talk about, ever.

For those of you who may be reading this and thinking, "Sure, that sounds fine for other people, but I still need to lose weight," I understand. I really do. What helps me when that thought pops up is this question: "What can I do to feel my best *today*?" Because even if I buy into the idea that I have to lose weight, my starting point for health and feeling good can't be when the weight is gone. The starting point is now, with how you feel and what you need today. Research from brilliant people like Dr. Kristin Neff[9] tells us that while we think what makes us into the people we want to be is buckling down and getting strict with ourselves, the opposite is actually true. The real root of the life we want starts with self-compassion. Which, conveniently, is also where body acceptance starts.

I believe this is also where lasting (meaning the conversation never ends) body acceptance comes from. It's living in and loving the body you have, and not making either of those dependent on something as mutable (again: because we're humans) as a number on a scale.

Bodies change. Weight changes. This is the process called life that we're all engaged in. So instead of a number, let the constant in your life be the sometimes lively, sometimes blah, sometimes transformative, sometimes mundane dialogue with yourself and your body.

Because nothing says "not giving up" like being willing to stay with yourself and be on your own side, applying kindness as often as possible.

It's important to acknowledge that body acceptance also doesn't mean that you'll never want your body to change.

I was chatting with a friend recently when she sheepishly mentioned something she wanted to change about her body.

"I don't know if I want to tell you," she squeaked out tentatively.

"It's fine; just tell me," I responded with a smile.

"But I feel conflicted about this change in some ways myself; it makes me feel like I might not be fully accepting of my body."

I laughed and said, "Who is?"

But I also followed up and said, "People get the mistaken idea that acceptance means you never change, but that couldn't be true even if we wanted it to be. Our bodies are always changing, so acceptance can never be a static thing."

I believe deeply that acceptance is always shifting, at least a little, because so are we; to me, that's an indisputable fact. Every day, things about our bodies are changing. Some are imperceptible (like what's happening on a cellular level). Some we know about but don't register most of the time (like hair growing, skin cells shedding, and so on). And some are things about our bodies that we might want to change.

For example, you might want to move your body more because it feels good (hello, walk I took this morning on a beautiful day!). You might shift what you eat from season to season because your body is craving something different (nothing is less appealing to me than salad in winter, but in summer, I eat it almost every day). You might want to make your body stronger or more flexible so you can keep yourself resilient in the face of a potential fall (after years of falling constantly, I finally started working with the mobility in my feet and ankles, and now it happens much less often). You might also want to get help, support, or treatment for something going on with your body. For example, I go to acupuncture and take supplements for anxiety.

You might also want to lose weight. Many people who begin to encounter the concept of body acceptance do so while still trying to lose weight. I know this not only from talking to countless people but also from my own experience because I did, too! And you know what? That's fine. If you've been in the diet cycle for years and years, you can't wait for the day when you never have a desire to try another diet again before trying body acceptance, or that day may never come. Patterns you've built up over years—even decades for many of us—will not go away overnight.

So if you want to lose weight, don't let it be a reason why you can't start doing this practice. Use the attitude of curiosity we talked about in the last chapter to start noticing *why* instead. What beliefs and/or patterns underlie that desire that you could get curious about and question?

Body acceptance doesn't mean you never change. And HAES doesn't mean you'll never lose weight. Both do mean you put your focus on healthy behaviors (not just your weight), tune into your body's current needs and desires, and meet them based on moving, eating, and otherwise nourishing yourself in ways that work for *you* in ways that you have access to (because of course due to the intersecting forms of oppression we talked about earlier, we do not all have the same access to resources to support us in this endeavor). The point is finding what works for your body. Some people who do this lose weight, others gain weight, and others' weight stays the same.

Personally, over all my years of dieting, despite short periods of weight loss, my weight went up. This is true for *so many* dieters because this is how the body responds to deprivation, which is what dieting trains our bodies for.[10] Since practicing body acceptance and HAES, though, my weight has stabilized.

Sure, it's not what I'd once fantasized (which would never have been possible for my body anyway because that's not how I'm built). But what I've found is that I'm far happier and even healthier now than I used to be. Because now what I eat meets what I need/want in the moment. I have a regular movement practice, and I have freed up all the time and other resources I used to flush down the toilet on dieting for things I enjoy. Now, will this always be true for me? Of course not. My health, like everyone else's, will ebb and flow. Just like dieting, HAES is not a destination or a forward-moving-only train.

Because here's the thing: You can make anything a hammer over your own head. That can be as true if the hammer is a diet as if it's thinking there's an end point to body acceptance and that you'll never get "there" or you're not doing it "right," so you might as well give up.

The point isn't to get a new hammer. It's to put the hammer down.

And one of the best ways to do that is by affirming your body with kindness.

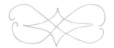

PRACTICES

Challenge What You Know on the Yoga Mat
(the Barometer)

One of the biggest ways I recognized the impact my yoga practice was having on my body and my life was by noticing how differently I felt both in and about my body over time.

So when I started teaching yoga, I wanted a way to offer a similar experience to students—helping them to notice what changed in their body and came into their awareness—within the context of one sixty- to ninety-minute class. And that's when I came up with the Barometer. (I'm surely not the only yoga teacher who does something similar; this is just what I call it.)

The idea is that you choose one pose or action (like lifting the arms overhead) to return to throughout a practice/class. This gives you the opportunity to both develop awareness of your body and see the benefits of the work you're doing in a very concrete way. I don't do this every class/practice, but I find it's nice to play with every few weeks.

What I love about the Barometer is that it gives you the opportunity to challenge what you know about poses you might be used to doing. By giving you a prolonged experience with the pose, you may discover all kinds of things about it, especially how best to make it work for your body. The Barometer is all about letting your internal experience of a pose guide you, rather than trying to put your body into a certain shape.

Here's an example of how it works (you could do this with any pose/action you'd like, though it needs to be one you can do an easeful version of with no warm-up, so keep it simple):

* Barometer pose: Down Dog with a chair (see the appendix for a description).

* Before you do any warm-up, do the Barometer pose. This gives you a sense of your body as you're starting the practice. Take a few deep breaths and then focus your attention on one or two body parts (for example, shoulders and hips). Ask yourself: What differences do I notice side to side in my shoulders? And hips? Where do I feel free? Less free? When you're done with those inquiries, make a mental note, because you'll be returning to this later.

* From here, continue into your warm-up, concentrating particularly on your focus areas (in this case, shoulders and hips).

* After the warm-up, come back to the Barometer, noticing any differences in your hips, shoulders, and body as a whole. You can ask the same questions as above, noting what differences, if any, you experience. As you go along, be alert to the following and ask yourself: Did you find the most freedom in your body after the hip work or the shoulder

work? Or was it a combo of both? This is a good way for you to learn more about your body as well as the pose you chose as your Barometer.

* Next continue into some standing poses, maybe concentrating on lengthening the spine and freeing the shoulders. Then it's back to the Barometer, more standing poses, and another Barometer to wrap up before cool-down/relaxation.

* In the last Barometer, again observe: What differences do you notice from the first time you did the pose?

* End with a cool-down and *Savasana*, as you'd like.

This technique can be used in many different ways, including with different poses (you can choose more or less complex poses, depending on what's right for your body) and actions. You could also do more or fewer check-ins, depending on your intention for the day and time available. Regardless of what you choose, the beauty of the Barometer is in how it focuses you very concretely on what is happening in your body and practice. This is a go-to for me when I'm feeling especially disconnected from myself.

Knowing how you feel in your body is also helpful for discovering what you need in your yoga practice. We're going to get into those details next.

Challenge What You Know Off the Yoga Mat

Using some of the general topics discussed in this chapter, consider what beliefs you have to challenge in your own life regarding your body. In addition to spending some time thinking about that, I like to take advantage of opportunities that are already present. For example, if I find myself thinking in "always" or "never" terms about my body, it's a great opportunity to check in and challenge. That shows up in thoughts like "I never want to do that pose again" or "I always mess up when it comes to my body." While it's entirely possible you may not enjoy a pose or want to do it again, statements like those warrant challenging just to see if, and in what ways, they're actually true today or if they're remnants of past stories (like the latter example).

Other opportunities to challenge off the yoga mat come when you're presented with a friend's latest diet, the latest "health" trend on TV, or an article forwarded to you from your cousin about the "5 best ways to lose weight this season." If you're anything like me, you feel a little quickening in your heart when you run into those things. "Oh," I think, before I can catch myself, "Is this what I've been waiting my whole life for?" Any time I think something like that, I know it's time to challenge those thoughts. Because is this diet or "health" plan or "detox" any different than the thousands before it? Of course not. Noticing your own patterns of belief help you build in automatic challenges and bring yourself back to center and your practice of presence, get curious, challenge, and affirm.

Inquiry

Inner observation isn't possible without the process of inquiry. Whenever I feel stuck in knowing how I feel (that is, most of the time), I ask myself a series of questions. Some of my favorites include:

* **Where am I in space?** This is less philosophical than it sounds. All it means is where am I in the room? Are my feet on the floor or tucked up? What are my back and hips in contact with if I'm sitting? What's the quality of light in the room? All these things help me get present so I can look a bit more deeply into my current experience.

* **What do I need?** Sometimes the answer is complicated, but more often than not it's quite simple—to move, drink some water, take a break, go outside, have a snack.

* **How can I meet that need in this moment, with what's available to me now?** This helps when the answer is "a vacation" and I don't have a plane ticket, money, time off, or a hotel reservation.

If you're new to this process, answering these questions may feel impossible, or you may be sure you're not getting the "right" answer to each one. So let me tell you this: There is no right answer. But I have a feeling you knew that already; our brains just don't always want to believe it. Also, keep in mind that this gets easier over time.

Not getting an answer or not being sure of it isn't a sign of failure. It's a sign of engagement.

All you're looking for in this process is information, and not knowing what you're finding is also information. Because a huge component of body acceptance is being in conversation with your body on a regular basis, these questions are like conversation starters you might look up before a first date. At first, they act as scaffolding. Later, you may be able to finish each other's sentences and not need them, but they helped you get from A to B.

ASK

your body

WHAT

do I need

IN

this moment

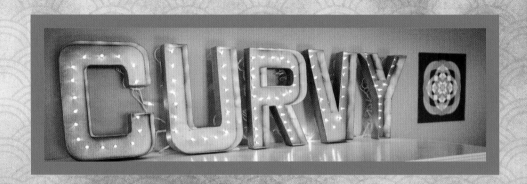

Affirm

Trust Me, This Is Way More Practical Than It Sounds

The primary way I learned the importance of making yoga work for you is through all the years I spent not knowing how to do that. One of the most vivid times I remember this happening is the first time I tried to get myself into Plow Pose, an often awkward and certainly challenging yoga pose. I was young (read: more willing to throw my body into any shape I could), so when the teacher said to rock forward from lying down on our backs, then swing our legs back over our heads, I did.

I didn't have time to be shocked by the outcome, though, because I was too overwhelmed by what I thought was my surely impending death. I hadn't realized until that moment that my teacher must have been contracted to put a hit on me and make it look like it was all my fault—because, yep, my boobs were about to strangle and/or suffocate me to death.

Trying to quietly gasp (two words that definitely do *not* go together) for breath, unsure of how many seconds I had left until my imminent demise, I lowered myself down and out of the pose. I certainly couldn't afford to wait until the teacher cued us out!

Once I came down and I reassured myself that I could, indeed, still take a few deep breaths, I just lay there, unsure of how to process what had just happened. This couldn't be the way the pose is supposed to feel, right? But everyone else was still there, seemingly serene (and I didn't hear anyone else barely clinging to life like I had been).

So I did the only logical thing: I blamed myself. (After convincing myself this probably wasn't a grand conspiracy after all.)

Because when you struggle in a yoga pose, and no one says anything to you directly, or even generally suggests some issues you might run into and how to address them, most of us are conditioned to blame ourselves.

But it doesn't have to be this way. You can equip yourself with tools to make the yoga poses work for you.

No life-flashing-before-your-eyes moments required.

And while the practice of yoga has been one of body acceptance for me over time, I was surprised to learn that the physical practice of the poses isn't the only component of yoga that supports body acceptance.

The Eight Limbs of Yoga and Body Acceptance

We've already talked about the *koshas*, which is one way the system of yoga teaches us about how to connect more with our bodies. Another perspective comes to us through *The Yoga Sutras*, a text in which the author, Patanjali, distilled the prevailing yoga wisdom of the time. (Scholars disagree on when Patanjali lived, but most estimate sometime between 500 BCE and 200 CE).[1] One of the things he delineates is the process of how yoga unfolds, which is known as the Eight Limbs of Yoga.

These limbs, or components, include what many of us picture when we think of yoga today: the poses. But that's just one part (and not even the first or last!) out of eight. The rest fill in a deeper picture, which links us back to ourselves: our body, our heart, our mind, our breath, and our connection with the universe. Luckily for those of us needing some help with body acceptance (aka pretty much all of us), this is exactly what we need.

In short, here are the Eight Limbs and how I think we can consider them in relation to body acceptance. It's important to note that though it doesn't always seem this way with how yoga is often represented these days, yoga didn't originate with white people in the West. It has a long history with roots in South Asia and a lineage that branches out to many different teachers, styles, and places around the world. One way we can honor that history is by acknowledging it and talking about how yoga has affected us rather than speaking broadly on behalf of yoga.

So what I have here is not a strict translation; you'd need a Sanskrit scholar for that, which definitely isn't me. This also isn't the end-all be-all way of thinking about the Eight Limbs. What I have here is how I think about these things in the context of body acceptance because yoga is more than just the poses, and I think it's valuable to consider how other parts of the practice may help us get to know ourselves and our bodies better.

Here they are:

1. *Yamas*

These are the ethical principles of yoga, including *ahimsa* ("compassion"—which must start with ourselves), *satya* ("truth"—first about who we are and then what we need), *asteya* ("nonstealing"—particularly, taking responsibility for what's yours, including how you feel), *brahmacharya* ("using your energy wisely"—pausing before acting, particularly on your own behalf), and *aparigraha* ("nonattachment"—trusting the process and letting go).

Let's break these down a little in relation to a closer relationship with your body.

Ahimsa—Compassion

I love that we start with compassion. How fitting! While this is often discussed in relation to other beings, many teachers share how it ultimately has to begin with ourselves. We have examples of how this works in yoga and meditation; for example, loving-kindness meditation. In loving-kindness meditation, we start by extending loving-kindness toward ourselves, and then we gradually send that love to a loved one, a neutral person (like an acquaintance), someone with whom we have difficulty, and then all beings everywhere.

In some traditions, though, until you can truly send love to yourself, you don't go any further. You continue practicing love toward self until you feel ready and able to move on to others. What a heart-opening contrast to how many of us often spend our days: giving, giving, giving to others until there's either nothing left for us or until we're so tired we don't have time to even notice how depleted we are, which isn't good for us or anyone else.

This also applies to the physical practice on the mat. There, *ahimsa* looks like being in dialogue with your own body. It also looks like using a prop. Finding the version of the pose that works for you. Asking for help. Noticing your breath. Not pushing yourself to the point of pain—physical, emotional, or mental.

Satya—Truth

It's amazing how closely connected telling the truth is with compassion, isn't it? In my yoga practice, this looks like allowing myself to discover and stay with the current truth of my body. That means not pushing myself into poses that were available for me at eighteen but aren't today (so hard!). It also means challenging myself to try something new when it's safe for my body but my mind is resisting (also hard!). In addition, it means acknowledging and accommodating injuries, making space for my curves and not beating myself up about it, and more things in this vein.

This concept also applies to my relationship with my body, particularly in the ongoing conversation with it that body acceptance asks for. Because if body acceptance is neither passive nor free from change like we talked about earlier, it for sure requires truth.

Asteya—Nonstealing

In relation to body acceptance, the most prominent thing to me about *asteya* is not stealing from myself. I've stolen so much of my own energy, time, and money while hating my body. When I look back at all that loss, it makes me so sad. But it also makes me grateful to be putting those resources to better use now.

The other thing I think of here is not stealing from other people in terms of making comparisons. On the surface, comparison may not seem like stealing from others, but I think it is. You're taking who they are and using it as a weapon against yourself—and possibly against them, too. By not doing this, we let people inhabit their bodies without judgment. And when we create the space for others to be who they are, and be okay in the body they have, we create the opportunity for us to do the same for ourselves.

Brahmacharya—Using Your Energy Wisely

While traditionally the energy referred to here is sexual, I think it's useful to consider wise use of all of our energy. Perhaps you've had this (or a similar) experience on your body acceptance journey: You have all good intentions of listening to your body, but then you wake up one day and realize—oof!—you're back in your old habits of body loathing.

Interestingly, I don't think the energy spent in body loathing is the waste in this context (though, of course, it's certainly not helpful) because this ebb and flow is just part of the process. The waste shows up in what often comes next, which I suspect could sound familiar to some of us (she says while raising her hand): berating yourself for being loathsome in the first place. How much time have you spent doing this? And does it ever encourage you to recultivate a relationship with yourself? I don't know about you, but whenever I try to boot camp myself into taking better care of and being kinder toward my body, it never works. I think a better use of our energy is to acknowledge where we are, that this isn't a sign of failure, and move forward from there.

Aparigraha—Nonattachment

There have been more times than I can count in my body acceptance journey that I thought I'd finally "gotten it." "Hooray!" I'd think. "Now I can move on from this whole body acceptance thing into more important parts of my life." Except—oops. Of course I wasn't done—far from it. I'd just come to another leg of the journey. *Aparigraha* helps me anchor into the beauty of process, not grasping onto a particular state of being but rather opening to whatever comes next.

2. Niyamas

These are the codes for how we should live, including *saucha* ("purity"— clarifying what we no longer need to get to the root of who we are), *santosha* ("contentment"—not false happiness, but being present with what is), *tapas* ("discipline"—in a way that feels really *good*), *svadhyaya* ("self-study"—my personal favorite because it asks us to continue to increase our capacity for self-awareness), and *isvarapranidhana* ("let go and let the divine in"—dropping into the wholeness of your body and its synergy with the universe). Let's unpack these.

Saucha

Saucha is usually translated as "purity," and I admit to being a bit squeamish about that idea. I think it's too easy for many of us today to think that we need to be modern-day ascetics in order to be spiritual, live up to society's expectations (hello, "detox" diets), and overall be good people.

Not too surprisingly, I don't buy that. Yoga is a clarifying practice. It helps us know what best serves our bodies, minds, and spirits and what doesn't. This is an essential component of body acceptance as we learn the movement, thoughts, beliefs, and actions that support us.

Santosha

Santosha is translated as "contentment," and I feel a big exhale of relief when I hear that. What is typically meant by this isn't that you're happy all the time, but rather that you can stay with your present experience. Another word I think of to describe this is "equanimity."

To me, this is body acceptance in a nutshell. It's being with your body as it is, relaxing into the truth of the present moment.

Tapas

Tapas is often translated as "heat" or "discipline," but I prefer Donna Farhi's translation of "burning enthusiasm."[2] I find discipline to be a counterproductive concept for many of us, due to its often harsh connotations, especially for those of us with any history of body image problems or disordered eating (and who among us can't raise our hand for that, right?). Most of us already have plenty of practice in being hard on ourselves.

I like to think of *tapas* as what keeps us connected to both yoga and body acceptance, especially when it feels hard. It's the process of showing up for yourself, your body, and your practice on a regular basis, returning to it with gentleness when you don't, and knowing that life is lived in the in between.

Svadhyaya

Okay, now we've come to my very favorite *niyama*! *Svadhyaya* means "self-study," and I think this is where things get *really* good in terms of the path yoga lays out for body acceptance.

In my experience, yoga helped me not only to begin to feel what was happening in my body, but also to be able to use that information going forward. So, for example, if I start to notice that I'm feeling anxious, I now know I can check in with my body to see where I feel it, which then gives me the opportunity to shift it. And the reverse is true, too—if I'm feeling good, why? Knowing what got me there may help me do something similar in the future.

Svadhyaya is the tool that helps us figure out what's up in the first place— and also helps us determine what to do about it (if anything).

Isvarapranidhana

I think of *isvarapranidhana* as the "let go and let the divine" of yoga—where you determine what the divine means to you. This can sometimes feel a bit complicated or unclear, though, particularly depending on how you relate to the concept of the divine (or don't). So (surprise, surprise) I think one way we can find our way in is through a bodily feeling of integration or peace within ourselves and our place in the universe.

You might find this while lying in *Savasana*. Or looking at the stars at night. Or in companionable silence with a long-time friend. Or watching your child play. Or swimming in the ocean. I've even felt it at times when I make a choice to be kinder to my body than I know I would have in the past.

3. Asana

These are the yoga poses, or what many of us think of when we think of yoga. But by having *asana* in the middle of the path, and closer to the beginning than the ending, we find a powerful lesson: It's the effect and benefit of the poses, not what poses you can do, that matter.

The yoga poses allow us to do the practice we've been discussing in this book—presence, get curious, challenge, and affirm—because they give us a clear time and embodied opportunity to do so. This is extremely helpful, particularly if you're new(er) to this process and getting started in your everyday life feels overwhelming. Starting on your yoga mat gives you a chance to practice, and what I've found is the more people do that, the more intentionally they're able to do so off the yoga mat, as well.

4. Pranayama

This is breath practice, so it's about building the bridge between the mind and the body. By tuning into the breath, even just once, we can come back to ourselves, back to our bodies, whenever we want.

There are many breath practices, but I think this one is the simplest and most profound because it can be done anytime, anywhere.

5. *Pratyahara*

This is withdrawal of the senses—but not from the world. It's being so grounded within yourself that you can listen to your own wisdom at any time. For example, sometimes when I'm feeling stressed and my to-do list is filling up way faster than my done list, I veg out in front of the TV while also surfing the web from my phone. Who doesn't, right? Usually, though, that level of sensory input is too much to help me feel relaxed, much less centered. But that's what *pratyahara* can do—it encourages us to slow down, to do one task at a time, rather than five. Or to make time to sit quietly with a cup of tea, without doing or listening to anything else. This is also what happens as we slow our bodies and lie down for *Savasana*. Usually the teacher will dim the lights and quiet the room, both of which better prepares us for rest and being with ourselves.

6. *Dharana*

This is concentration, or single-minded focus. In relation to body acceptance, *dharana* is a wonderful opportunity to focus on a particular feeling you want to cultivate, like body neutrality, if not acceptance or love. One great way you might practice this is by finding something to focus on when you're feeling bad about your body. For instance, when you get into a negative place, it often feels overwhelming and as if one negative thought is spiraling into another and another. To switch gears, shift your focus to your breath. Make contact with the physical sensation of the breath entering in and exiting out through the nostrils. Through this focus on a neutral action in your body, you're more likely to shift back into a more neutral attitude toward your body, too.

7. *Dhyana*

Ah, meditation. Notice how we didn't get here until now? Once we've moved our bodies and quieted and focused our minds, we're ready for the wide mind of meditation—where we take in everything about ourselves and our world, not necessarily without judgment, but letting whatever thoughts surface, including judgment, pass by without attachment, perhaps using the practice we've been discussing—presence, get curious, challenge, and affirm.

8. *Samadhi*

This is bliss or enlightenment, but it's not a once-and-done kind of deal. Rather, once you find a feeling of oneness with the universe, the intention is to come back to the world as you know it—with what you now know about how infinite and amazing we each are.

In body acceptance, these are fleeting moments when I feel happy and whole in my body and sense my rightful place in the universe. I experience this most reliably when I'm taking a deep breath by the ocean, but it could happen anywhere.

Using the Eight Limbs as a blueprint, you may find a way into the practice of presence, get curious, challenge, and affirm—as well as into yourself.

And since one of the main doorways is often the yoga poses, or *asanas*, all you need are some tools to practice in a way that works for you, no matter what your body shape or size, and without the need to put your leg behind your head. Because, goodness knows, I won't, at least not without a trip to the hospital!

Let's get into it.

Curvy Alignment

The process of figuring out how to make yoga poses work for you starts with figuring out what you need. It also starts with knowing and accepting that what you need and how your pose looks will be different from that of other people.

The first time I saw a picture of myself in a yoga pose, I was shocked. As in, completely flabbergasted. All this time I'd thought I was aligned, but when I looked at the photo, I thought my knee looked locked and that my hip was completely misaligned.

So I came into the pose again, building it up bit by bit in front of a mirror to confirm. And that's when it hit me: What I'd seen as misalignment was actually just the shape of my body. Because I was used to seeing straight lines and angles in yoga books, which are usually full of very thin people (if not outright skeletons), as well as on my teachers whose bodies were very different from mine, I hadn't realized how different a yoga pose looked on my body.

What a revelation.

With this in mind, let's talk through some things to look out for to ensure that you are practicing safely and comfortably for your body. What I've included here are options that can be useful for curvy bodies that you might not see or hear in traditional yoga classes. By incorporating them into your routine, you can adapt the practice for yourself and know that you can participate in the classes you want. Not everyone will experience all (or any) of these issues, but I see them often enough that I think they're worth mentioning. Of course, it is always wise to consult a doctor or physical therapist before beginning any movement program. You might also like to consult an in-person yoga teacher to get more personalized information. For specific pose instructions, see the appendix, which includes more detailed information. If you're brand-new to yoga, don't worry if you don't yet know the poses by their names. You'll still get a good review of information to start your practice, and you can always return here later once you're more familiar.

Foundation/Feet

One way to begin building the alignment of a yoga pose is from its foundation. In seated poses, that's the sit (sitz) bones (or the bones that you're sitting on, also called the "ischial tuberosities"). In standing poses, it's the feet.

Sometimes in yoga you will hear teachers talk about the four corners of the feet, meaning pressing down underneath the root of the big toe, the root of the pinky toe, and the two sides of the heel. Most of us do not naturally think of the heel as having two sides, though, so I prefer to consider the three points of the feet, which creates a triangle of support.[3] You can look at or visualize the bottom of the foot and imagine pressing down on the ball of the foot directly underneath the big toe and the pinky toe, as well as the center of the heel to understand this.

Starting with the triangle of support under both feet is a good way to begin and can help you judge if you need to make any adjustments to your stance.

If your feet have a tendency to roll in or out, you will need to be extra aware of the triangle of support. Sometimes it's hard to know if you have this pattern or not, though. One way to find out is to stand the way you regularly stand, as if you were waiting in line at the grocery store. As you do, observe the triangle of support (or lack thereof!) under both feet. It's very likely that you naturally press down under some parts of the foot but not others. We all have these patterns in our bodies.

Your feet may roll in or out due to injury, genetics, or a number of other factors. In addition, your feet may roll in or out as your body's response to creating a base of support that works for you. Each of us needs a base of support that is appropriate for our own body. The only issue arises when your body does that on its own without your awareness, so your feet end up rolling out, rather than you taking a slightly wider stance with grounded feet (which just means the feet are engaged in the triangle of support). If your feet roll in or out, you may have a tendency to get light or not press down at all under at least one of the three points of the triangle of support, so your job is to return your light awareness there whenever you notice it not pressing down and reengage. Grounding your feet can keep you stable in your poses and can also help you build strength in your feet and ankles to keep you safe both on and off the mat. Grounding your feet does not mean mashing your feet down (and probably locking your knees in the process). It just means feeling the feet fully in contact with the floor.

If you have any type of foot pain (plantar fasciitis, heel spurs, swelling, and the like), consider taking a shorter stance in wide-legged standing poses (such as Warrior 2, Side Angle, and Triangle). Sometimes the feet can get cramps in standing poses because they're trying to do all the work of keeping your body upright. So whether you're feeling discomfort in the feet for one of the reasons stated above or another reason, experiment with a slightly shorter stance. You can do this by moving the feet in half an inch to an inch (1.3 cm–2.5 cm), checking in, then adjusting your stance as needed. This may give you the stability you need to build awareness, strength, and mobility in other areas of the body that can help support you even more. This can be a bridge while those things develop. You might also alternate between front- (Warrior 1, Tree, Pyramid) and side-facing standing poses to give the feet some variety in the work they have to do.

Knees

If I had to name the number one complaint I hear from my students of every shape and size, it's knees. Pain in the knees usually shows up in two primary forms in yoga classes: pain when moving and pain when kneeling.

Pain When Moving:

When moving into standing poses where the knee is bent (such as Warrior 1, Warrior 2, or Side Angle), go slowly. I like to encourage dynamic movement here, which means moving with your breath. Dynamic movement allows you to move and challenge your body within the context of an already aligned pose. For example, in Warrior 1 you can bend/straighten your front leg a few times in alignment, moving with your breath. That process can allow you to warm up your knee a bit before holding it, as well as help you find where the best place for you to hold it today will be.

As you go along with the pose, be sure to check in with your back foot and find the triangle of support underneath it. With the back leg helping, rather than being unengaged, you can provide an anchor for the front leg, which helps stabilize the knee, as well as the whole body.

Another thing to try, as a way to support the knees in standing poses, is a different instruction. It's amazing the difference language can make in our bodies sometimes! So after you go through the bending/straightening process above, take a short break and do another pose. Then return to the one you were in before and try this (allowing your hips and torso to come along for the ride): Inhale and move your thigh forward, keeping your back thigh stable; exhale and straighten your leg. Repeat this several times at the pace of your own breath.

If you're reading that and thinking, "Huh?," you're definitely not alone. While "Move your thigh forward" isn't language you might be used to, give it a try. What happens when you move your thigh forward is that your knee naturally starts to bend. As you try it, ask yourself the questions from above again: "Where does it feel like this movement originates?" And "What sensation, if any, do I feel in my knee?"

Some people will not experience a difference with the language variation. But it's not uncommon, especially for people with knee concerns, to feel as if the movement originates closer to the hip (not the knee) when they're moving their thigh forward as opposed to bending their knee, and that they therefore experience less sensation/pain in their knee.

If that instruction was useful for you, just mentally instruct yourself to "Move the thigh forward" when your teacher says, "Bend your knee" to give that same support for your knee. What's happening here is that you're engaging your quadriceps (the top of your thigh) to help stabilize the knee. But sometimes the word "engage" can be even more confusing an action to make than "Move the thigh forward," which is why I prefer the latter. What's most important, though, is that you support your joints well, so use whatever language works for you!

Pain When Kneeling:

If you have pain in kneeling poses, you have a few options. (1) Don't do them. Seriously: There are plenty of other good choices, so why risk something as valuable as your knee? (2) If you're pretty much okay on your knees but just don't like the feeling of your knee digging into the hard ground, try placing a blanket or a knee pad under your knee and see if that helps. (3) Do the pose in a different way. For example, if a kneeling pose is being taught, see how you could do it from a seated position or lying down instead. Sometimes changing the orientation to the floor is all that's needed. Here are some examples for common kneeling poses:

* Cat/Cow (*Chakravakasana*): Instead of doing this from kneeling on hands and knees (also called Tabletop position), try it from a comfortable seated position (legs crossed or extended—or in a chair). (There's more on this in the appendix).

* Gate (*Parighasana*): From a seated position, tuck your left leg in toward your pelvis (if you're in a chair, simply leave your left leg where it is); extend your right leg out to the right. Place your right hand on your right leg and begin sliding your hand down your leg, not collapsing onto your right side. When you get to a point where you feel the side collapse, stop. Now rotate your left shoulder up and back, extending your left arm out over your left ear.

* Camel (*Ustrasana*): From a seated position, place the hands on the backs of the hips, fingertips pointing down (hands could also grip the sides of the chair back if you're in a chair). Inhale and lift your sternum; exhale and roll your shoulders back. The same can be done from standing, with the front body in light contact with the wall.

No matter what the kneeling pose is, if you're looking for an alternative, ask yourself (or your teacher!) this question: "What is the benefit of this pose?" When you understand the general action and intention of the pose, it becomes simpler to come up with an alternative by adding support and/or moving the pose in relation to gravity (that is, shifting it from seated to lying down, from lying down to standing, and so on).

Legs

One of the foundational poses of yoga is Mountain, or *Tadasana*. It's often taught with feet together or, at the most, hip-distance apart. However, because of flesh around the thighs, this position (especially with feet together) can be uncomfortable at best and unsafe at worst for some people. For example, if I stand with my feet together, my knees buckle out due to the compression of the skin around my thighs. Throwing my body out of alignment to conform to a narrow (literally) idea of a pose is not a good idea! If the same is true for you, scrap it!

Instead, try this experiment: Stand with your feet as close together as possible and observe the following: Are you able to press down onto the triangle of support under both feet? Where do you feel stable? Or unbalanced? Do you have the ability to rock slightly forward and back, side to side, without feeling like you're going to topple over?

Once you have a sense of yourself with feet together, try the same experiment as above with feet hip-distance apart, meaning the distance between the internal hip bones. This is usually much narrower than you may think because we're not talking about the outer flesh of your hips, but rather the internal hip bones, which, for most people, are a few inches (roughly 7 cm) on either side of your belly button and down an inch or two (2–5 cm or so) (of course, precise measurements will differ for each person). Again, get a sense of how you feel here and ask yourself the questions above.

Finally, try this experiment: Begin to slowly and gradually step your feet a tiny bit further apart until you find a comfortable distance for you. You want to find the position closest to hip-distance apart that works for you so your skeleton can help support you. A comfortable distance apart means that you feel both stable and as if you have at least a little room to move (mostly, that you just don't feel squeezed like a tube of toothpaste). You may find that the comfortable position is one of the ones you've already tried.

But if you observe that it's different in some way (as I do—I like to be just a smidge wider than hip-distance apart), make a note of the difference so that you can return to that position any time you come back to Mountain Pose. Many people who find hip distance a bit too narrow will find comfort and stability with just a little bit more space. With a Mountain Pose that works for you, you will end up doing many other standing poses (particularly the front-facing ones) with greater ease because you're starting with the base of support that is right for you. And when seated, the same is true: Find your comfortable leg-distance apart and work from there. We're not talking about going so wide that your body can't support you safely, but just giving yourself the freedom of taking up the space you need.

Wrists

Wrists are delicate and finicky creatures. And they can cause some discomfort in yoga poses—especially poses with an arm balance component like Downward-Facing Dog (Down Dog). If your wrists are giving you any trouble in a pose like that, here are a few things to try. (1) Roll up the front edge of your mat and place the roll under the heel of your hand, with your fingertips forward, touching the ground. This can take a little pressure off the wrists. (2) Use a yoga wedge (easily purchased online or in some yoga-specific shops) to do the same thing. (3) Make fists with your hands and do the pose on your fists (bottom of the hand on the ground, not the knuckles). (4) Holding onto three- or five-pound (1.5–2-kg) dumbbells can create a similar effect to option 3 but may be easier on the hands for some people because the dumbbell is bearing the pressure into the floor. (5) Depending on the pose, you may be able to come onto the forearms, instead of the wrists. (6) Do another variation of the pose, perhaps with the wall or a chair, that may involve less wrist pressure.

Booty/Bum/Butt/Bottom

Whatever you call it, the shape/size of yours may make it difficult to lie on your back comfortably. These poses can cause your upper back and neck to get crunched, as well as your lower back. That's because the flesh of the bum is causing your spine not to lie down in accordance with its natural curves (yes, even the spine has curves!). This is particularly relevant in *Savasana*, or the final relaxation pose of most yoga classes, where you're often instructed to lie flat on your back with your legs extended and your arms resting by your sides.

Our goal here is to lengthen the spine from the tailbone end, neck end, and/or lower back in order to bring more comfort and freedom. You can choose from several options here. (1) Take your *Savasana* in a different position that you find more comfortable (even a different restorative pose!). (2) Begin with your knees bent, feet flat on the floor. Step your feet an inch (2.5 cm) or so closer toward your hips so you can press down under the triangle of support under both feet. Press through your feet to lift your hips up just enough to tuck your tailbone slightly. You can also bring your hands to the backs of your hips and move the skin down toward your feet as you do this, then setting your hips back down. This small action can lengthen your lower back. (3) Place a blanket or the rolled-up top of your mat under your head; this is sometimes enough to align the neck and shoulders more comfortably. (4) If that wasn't enough or you don't have something to put under your head, gently lift your head and bring your hands to the ridge of your skull. From here, lightly tuck your chin toward your chest, then set your head back down. Doing this with the head lifted is preferable to just tucking the chin with the head down because you can get a little more length in your neck, which can help free up the lower back. (5) Put a bolster, a rolled-up blanket, or the rolled-up edge of your mat under your knees to release your lower back. (6) Do some combination of all of these that works for you. Feel free to use these tips in any supine (lying on the back) poses that you'd like.

Belly

I think the belly is the area that makes most people most uncomfortable—physically but also emotionally. We're not usually taught to acknowledge, much less touch, our bellies!

I usually recommend two things to give bellies a little more space: (1) Step your feet wider, and (2) move the belly skin. Stepping your feet wider works well in standing poses (such as Standing Forward Bend) and seated poses (such as Seated Forward Bend). When the feet are too narrow in these positions, the belly can feel stuck, or compressed, by the legs. Stepping the feet wider can reduce or eliminate this issue. This is what we talked about in the previous section on Mountain Pose.

As we discussed there, move the feet out gradually and gently until you find a position that works for you. If you do step the feet wide in a Standing Forward Bend, be sure to lightly draw your navel toward your spine, engage your quadriceps, and bend your knees when coming back up (this is actually good to do in general—it's just especially true when the feet are wider apart, perhaps even stepping the feet back in if you'd gone quite wide).

Moving the belly skin itself is also a radically awesome option. It's radical not only because it works so well but because it gets you in touch (literally) with your belly, which is something very few of us do. The less we ignore whole parts of ourselves, the easier it becomes to accept our wholeness.

Though we rarely receive this message, it's absolutely okay to touch your own belly, your own body. Make yourself comfortable in the poses so you can create and continue a yoga practice that works for you. Nothing will make you quit yoga faster than forcing your body into positions that don't work for you!

There are several options for making space for your belly, depending on the pose and your belly: (1) Lift the belly up, (2) move the belly down, and/ or (3) move the belly a little to the middle. I personally prefer a combination of these three, but I've come to find that it's largely a matter of personal preference (as well as what pose we're talking about). I say whatever floats your boat is A-OK!

You can read more about how to do these options in the appendix. In a nutshell, though, it's about as easy as it sounds: Place your hands on either side of your belly, closest to your hips. Either hold the belly and move it up, laying it back down once you come into position; press it in and move it down toward your pelvis; or move it to the middle. Whatever you choose, remove your hands once you move the belly and voilà! You now have a little more room to move comfortably into your pose.

When you lift the belly up, you are creating space in the juncture between the hip and the belly, allowing the hip to close more, thus often coming into the pose a bit further and more comfortably, though more skin may now be in front of you. When you tuck the belly down, the opposite happens. Now the hip may have a little less space to close, but you have less skin in front of you, which can feel more comfortable and also possibly allow you to come forward a bit more. When you move the skin to the middle (especially in twists), you are making space on the side of the body where you are moving. Too often, curvy people are pegged as inflexible in classes when, in reality, we just need to adjust the pose to our bodies and then figure out where we really are in the pose.

Chest/Breasts

Ah, the dreaded death-by-boob smush. This shows up most often in inversions, and it can happen for people of all gender identities and expressions. There are a few things you can do for this. (1) Take a less upright inversion. The more up-and-down the position, the higher the likelihood for chest strangulation/suffocation. (2) Create space in the back of your neck in poses like Legs Up the Wall by slowly and gently lifting your head off the ground an inch or so, tucking your chin, and lowering your head back down (in supine positions, only do this in poses where you're lying fully on your back, like Legs Up the Wall—not Bridge, Shoulderstand, or Headstand). This technique also works in poses like Downward-Facing Dog, which we don't always think of as an inversion, but it is. There, take a moment to lengthen the spine. With the spine lengthened, tuck your chin to your chest, then lower the spine back down. This can feel counterintuitive, but creating the space in the back of your neck allows you to be in the pose more comfortably, even if your face is closer to your chest than before. (3) Fight gravity: This is something I learned from Megan Garcia.[4] How this works is by making a loop with a strap and putting it on over your head, as you would a shirt. You then cinch the strap at the top of the chest, making it snug but not painfully tight. With this in place, it will help you fight gravity when you're in an inverted, or upside-down, position. (You can read more about this in the description for Bridge Pose in the appendix.) If that doesn't work, you can also try a different bra or a different pose. You can receive the benefits (and way less risk of strangulation) in Legs Up the Wall. That pose is a great way to experience the benefits of inversions, letting your body be in a different relationship to gravity than it usually is, but in an accessible, comfortable way.

Getting Up and Down from the Floor

I want to add a note here about one of the challenges of many yoga classes that is often not discussed: Getting up and down from the floor. Very few of us spend much time doing this in our everyday lives, so it makes sense that when we're asked to (especially multiple times) in yoga classes, it can be hard. If you know this is going to be an issue for you, I encourage you to mention it to your teacher ahead of time. The place where you're practicing may have a chair you can use to either sit in for the seated poses or to provide a stable base of support (as long as it doesn't have wheels!) to help you come up and down. If that isn't available, another option is to place your yoga mat very near a wall so that you can use the wall similarly to the chair. If the place where you're practicing has yoga blocks, you can use them in a similar way, too—bending forward from standing, placing your hands on the blocks, and then slowly bending one knee down and then the other (and doing the reverse when coming up to standing).

As you continue to experiment with these pose options, remember that you only have one goal: to see what's working in your body today. Some days that's clearer than others, but the more you try different options, the more comfortable you become with both the poses and where you are in your practice.

Finding *Your* Yoga

I really enjoy being told I'm awesome (who doesn't, right?). I like knowing that I'm growing, moving forward, and pushing myself. I used to be a total achievement hound, reveling in others' praise.

But here's the thing. Others' praise? It doesn't teach me all that much. It feels *really* good, but in terms of changing how I feel about myself or validating that I'm enough just as I am—well, that rarely comes from other people.

I'd venture to say that it never does. Even when I think it does, if I don't believe it myself, it makes no difference what others say about how good, talented, or far along in my practice I am.

So that's why I don't talk about levels when it comes to yoga. I know that people like to be told they're on level 3 (or 100, whatever your numbering system is) of a pose. And many of us nearly faint from happiness when we're told we're intermediate or advanced.

But I don't buy it for yoga—especially when it comes to the physical practice of *asanas*, or yoga poses. Just because someone can rock out a crazy arm balance on the edge of a cliff doesn't mean his practice is better or more advanced than someone who would never even consider trying that—or vice versa. There's nothing wrong with complex poses, and they can definitely be fun to experiment with sometimes, but they don't tell you anything more about the relationship you're cultivating with yourself than any other pose does.

Yoga is a vehicle for self-acceptance and internal transformation. So it doesn't matter if you get that via balancing on your nose or lying in *Savasana*. You get to choose what's helpful for you.

Sometimes when people hear about Curvy Yoga, they assume that curvy = easy. In fact, someone asked one of my students that very question at a place where I teach, and as she recounted the story to me, she laughed heartily. She said, "Ask my hamstrings if it's easy!"

We have an interesting relationship to challenge in our society. Many of us think of challenge as pushing us beyond what we thought was physically possible—even to the point of injury. We imagine that if we're not close to passed out on the floor, we haven't gotten a "good workout."

I'd say that nearly the opposite is true, though. It's not challenging to blindly do what someone is telling you and push past your body's signals; that's what many of us have been trained to do for a long time. What's challenging is listening to a teacher's guidance and checking it against your own experience. Working at a level that is most appropriate for you that day, which sometimes looks like doing a sweaty, vigorous practice and sometimes looks like taking *Savasana*, or Relaxation Pose, as your entire practice.

So I invite you to use your attention and intention to notice how you're moving along in your practice. You'll know if and when you're advancing without anyone outside of you telling you. You'll find more openness in your body and more receptivity in your life. You'll find renewed strength and balance on the mat and off.

The incredible thing is that the process of noticing is also a reward in and of itself. As you notice more, you wake up more to your life, bringing what you thought you wanted from others' praise—like validation and acceptance—but in tangible forms you can hold on to.

Because what's changed isn't others' ideas. What's changed is you.

How to Find a Body-Affirming Yoga Class

One of the most frequently asked questions I receive is how to find a curvy-friendly yoga class. I have a couple of answers for this: The first is to check out the list of Curvy Yoga–certified teachers on my website (www.curvyyoga.com, and we also have a virtual studio if that's more your style). There may just be someone in your area!

And the second (until we get a certified Curvy Yoga teacher in every town, which is definitely my goal) is how to find a teacher you like. Because when you're ready to try a yoga class, whether for the first time or the hundredth, it may be a little scary sometimes. What will it be like? How will you know what to do? Will you feel like part of the group? Will you be able to keep up?

The good news is that you don't have to go in with no information. You can use the following tips to find a teacher who meets your needs, regardless of whether she's Curvy Yoga–certified or not.

A great place to start is to figure out what your needs are. Take some time to do a thorough assessment; needs you weren't expecting may emerge if you give it some time. For example, I'll assume that you're looking for someone who is welcoming of curvy folks, so there's one need. Depending on your unique circumstances, others may include the ability to work with beginners, someone who can help you accommodate a particular injury/illness, friendliness, and/or whatever other things you're looking for.

With your needs list in hand, you can begin researching. Of course, the Internet is helpful for this task. Spend some time searching things like "yoga" and the name of your town. Ask your friends for recommendations. And, hold it all lightly enough so your gut instinct can emerge. Just because a teacher is beloved by some people doesn't mean he's right for you. It's possible the folks who love that teacher have different needs than you do. And vice versa. Just because some people don't like a particular teacher doesn't mean you won't.

In addition, be creative about where you look. Of course, yoga studios are a natural place to find yoga teachers. But yoga teachers abound these days, so you can also look at community centers, libraries, parks, schools, gyms, houses of worship, and any other place you think may offer yoga.

While the number of curvy-friendly yoga teachers continues to grow, there is still a dearth of us in most areas. So, in addition to looking for a Curvy Yoga class, here are some other possible keywords to look for if you are new to yoga: yoga for every body, gentle yoga, accessible yoga, welcoming yoga, hatha yoga, slow-flow yoga, and beginner's yoga. If you prefer a faster-paced class, you're likely to find words like vinyasa yoga or flow yoga. Any class can be a good fit for a curvy practitioner, depending on the needs list you came up with (although, if you're brand-new to yoga, I usually recommend a slower pace at first, just so you can get the hang of the poses and have more opportunities to ask questions).

I encourage you to compile a list of at least two or three potential teachers whose classes you'd like to try. Once you have their names and contact info, consider connecting with them before class. I love hearing from new students before they come to class; it is a great way to get to know them better and assuage any potential fears they may have. So when you reach out to them, be sure to share any questions/concerns you have. Here are a few you might consider (feel free to use or adapt):

* **What props are available in your class, and when/how do you incorporate them?** If a teacher uses props in her class, it gives me a clue that she is at least somewhat knowledgeable about adapting poses to her students' needs.

* **Do you offer pose modifications during class?** This gives the teacher a clue that you will want/need various pose options, and it will also give you a chance to hear more about the teacher's thoughts on that.

* **What is your experience teaching curvy-bodied students?** It's useful to hear that a teacher has taught curvy-bodied students in the past. If he says he doesn't have much experience but he does have experience modifying poses for a people with a number of different injuries, abilities, ages, and the like, that is also a good sign that he can help you come up with creative solutions. Although experience with curvy bodies is obviously helpful, I think the most important thing is for the teacher to have a spirit of willingness to help you find what works for you in a nonjudgmental atmosphere.

How they respond (hopefully helpfully and promptly) will give you more insight into whether or not you want to try their class. And when you show up in class, they will already know at least a little bit about you. Just be sure to remind them—"I'm Anna. We emailed the other day about class," so you can pick up the conversation from there.

It's almost always less stressful to try something new with a friend in tow, isn't it? As you're deciding on some classes to try, chat up the possibility with your friends. People are often game to try things like this—especially since they can go with you (and you've already done the legwork). So if having a friend with you would make you feel more comfortable, by all means make it a date!

Just like finding a new hairstylist, you don't always find the right teacher/class on the first try. So adopt an attitude of curiosity and try out a few classes. Aim to try ones at times that fit your schedule on a regular basis so you could go back if you like the class. And as long as you don't hate the class, consider trying it two or three times before making a final decision. Yoga teachers are like the rest of us; some days they're more "on" than others, so it's good to give them a fair shake.

Oftentimes, in a new class there is at least one thing you didn't "get" or wanted more information about. It can feel scary sometimes to ask about this, but I definitely encourage you to try anyway. Teachers usually love helping you figure out what is right for you, so if you have a follow-up question, ask! You'll continue connecting and building a relationship with the teacher. If you have lots of questions and/or need some in-depth help, ask the teacher if she offers private sessions. This is a great way to get what you need in a concentrated dose. You'll pay more than you would for a group class, but just a few private sessions can often get you the info you need to practice safely and well for you, whether in group classes or at home.

As your foray into classes continues, don't forget the most important step: checking in to see what your body is telling you. So if you get a weird vibe but aren't sure what it was about (as often happens because many of us doubt our first instinct), by all means double-check it and try the class again. But if it persists, trust your feeling. You want to find a yoga class where you feel comfortable and accepted; it's worth the time to find a class where that little inner voice isn't telling you something isn't right.

Hopefully, these steps will help you find a class you love! If not, though, it's time to reassess. Here are several options to consider: If you like the teacher but the class isn't quite right, get in touch with him and let him know what you're looking for. Many teachers offer several different styles of classes, so you may not have found the right class yet. If the teachers aren't a good fit, go back through the research steps and find a few more to try out.

The main thing I want you to know is that if one (or even more than one!) yoga class/style/teacher isn't for you, that doesn't mean that *yoga* isn't for you. It just means you haven't yet found the right fit. I find that keeping this in mind is *so* helpful because it keeps you out of the self-blame trap so many of us fall into and keeps you in the realm of curiosity and experimentation.

You have the right to body-affirming yoga that works for your body. And with the tools in this book, as well as the support of an in-person teacher, you can find just that!

Remember: The main key to making yoga work for you and using it as a tool for body acceptance is to approach the whole process with kindness.

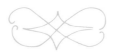

PRACTICES

Affirm Your Body on the Yoga Mat

Let your yoga practice be a time when you grow your ability to affirm your body in the moment. One way you can do this is as the conclusion to the practice we've been discussing—presence, get curious, challenge, and now affirm.

Here's what that could look like in one particular pose:

* Get present in your body: Feel your feet on the floor, bum on the floor, spine elongating, or whatever is relevant in the pose

* Get curious—ask one of the questions we talked about earlier, such as "What's happening with my breath here?"

* Challenge any negative thoughts, old stories or patterns that come up. For example, if you thought something like "Ugh, I'm not breathing again! What's wrong with me?," challenge that belief by moving into the next step.

* Affirm your body. So after finding a thought like the one above to challenge, give yourself permission to be human and right where you are. This could look like smiling, exhaling, and moving on. Or it could look like replacing the negative

comment with a more positive one, such as "I have a pattern of holding my breath, just like so many people do; this is an opportunity to breathe again."

Over the course of a yoga class (whether at home or in-person), you can repeat this process in various poses whenever you remember. Natural class transition times are easy ones to build into your process, such as when class starts, when you move from seated to standing (or vice versa), and before and after Savasana.

Another way to consider the practice in the context of a whole yoga class is to view each step moving along with you through all the poses, following the ebb of the class. So rather (or in addition to) applying the practice in individual poses, you apply it to the arc of the class. Here's what that might look like:

* When class is starting, get present in your body as above.

* As class proceeds, stay curious. Check in and ask yourself questions as they occur to you. The more you do this, the more organic that will become.

* When something worth challenging arises, do so.

* Throughout the practice, affirm your body and experience, making sure to do this very intentionally at the end of class as you transition into the rest of your day.

Affirm Your Body Off the Yoga Mat

Similar to what we just discussed about affirming your body on the yoga mat, you can apply the practice off the mat. Here's what that could look like in a given moment or experience (such as a time you find yourself feeling stressed, tired, down on yourself, or otherwise needing an opportunity to come back to your body):

∗ Presence yourself in your body. You can do this anywhere, anytime, and no one has to notice. All it requires is a moment (usually less than one minute, if even that!) to notice your body in space.

∗ Get curious about what's happening. If you're tired, ask yourself why or what you could do to shift your energy right now, with the resources you have on hand. If you're feeling down on yourself, get curious about what else is going on and how you might be able to support yourself.

∗ Challenge any negative thoughts, stories, beliefs that might be coming up.

∗ Affirm your body as it is, just in this moment. There is no need to change or become a new person. Who you are already is intrinsically enough.

Similarly to what we talked about on the yoga mat, you could also apply this practice over the course of a set period of time or a day (I wouldn't go longer than that; just start again the next day). Here's what that might look like:

* Before you get out of bed in the morning (or however soon you can after you rise), get present in your body.

* As your day proceeds, stay curious about what comes up. Whenever you notice how you're feeling physically or emotionally, use it as an opportunity to check in and ask yourself any relevant questions.

* When you do that, challenge any negative beliefs that come up.

* Before you move along with your day, affirm your body.

* Before you go to bed at night, affirm your body.

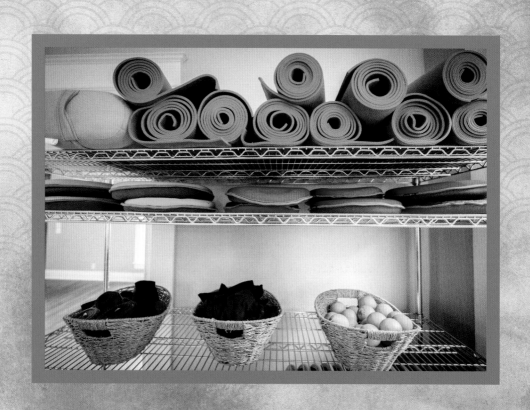

Practice

With Kindness, Again and Again

One of the first times I showed my body kindness was completely unintentional. I had no other choice.

When I was in graduate school, I lived alone. I'd never been happier in my life; I adored having my own space. It was everything Virginia Woolf said it would be. The only thing was that living alone did occasionally leave me susceptible to some bad late-night ideas.

One such bad late-night idea was buying my first bottle of Overnight Weight Loss pills. While I don't recall the actual name, it was only 2 percent less literal than this. I wish the name had been more subtle so I wouldn't seem so gullible, but as I've often told friends, if I'd ever been around a cult, I'm sure I would have been the first to join.

"Haven't been able to lose weight?!" the TV commercial boomed.

"That's because you've been sold a bill of goods and thought diets would work. But diets won't work because they don't utilize X chemical in your body that has recently been discovered to hold the key to quick and effortless weight loss while you sleep!"

I mean, it just made so much sense to me in that moment. You can see that, right?

In that moment, I had the fatal thought that has brought down so many: "How bad could it be?"

So I got out my credit card (also famous last words) and bought it.

I probably don't need to tell you that I got a second bottle free with purchase since I'd had the wisdom to be awake during this special, twenty-minute-only window. I felt pretty darn smug indeed and headed off to bed, grateful to know I had to waste my time "just" sleeping for only a night or two more. Soon, my sleep would be working for me.

I can still feel the bottle in my hand. It fit neatly into my palm when my fingers curled around it. It had a white label with blue lettering.

"Very elegant," I thought. "I like that it doesn't have to overdo it by being garish." As though something called Overnight Weight Loss weren't already way more garish than anything that has ever existed.

Though I felt proud inside that I'd made such a clever purchase, something still told me to stuff it in the back of a drawer where my then-boyfriend wouldn't see it. "Don't want him to know my secrets," I thought. As though anything less than shame could cause someone not only to hide something in the back of a drawer but also to cover it over with papers and other junk so it would never be found unless on purpose.

The first week of taking the pills was bliss. I strutted everywhere I went and got on the scale every day. Lucky me, I had one of those scales that ticked down a tenth of a pound at a time. So every day, a little smidge would be gone. And if it wasn't, I could feel it breaking free. I just knew it.

After the first week, I noticed my heart skipping a beat here or there. Though it was on my radar, I didn't think of it beyond a few seconds past when it happened. Been there, done that, I'd thought. This was hardly my first foray into weight loss drugs; I knew I just had to push through.

Another week passed, and I started to get angry that I wasn't sleeping well. It turns out that losing weight in your sleep is none too restful.

Nothing seemed right in my apartment. The A/C wasn't strong enough, and I still wasn't adjusted to the swampy Florida heat. My mattress was too hard. Or too lumpy, depending on where I rolled. And geez, why was life so intense?! Of course I couldn't sleep, I reassured myself, thinking of all these things lined up against me.

It took me a few days to realize that, no matter what I did, my heart wouldn't stop racing. And that it was like a record player ever so slowly starting to wear out, skipping beats. Not often. Just more often than before, which was never.

After another week or so, I suspected the pills and thought I should be reasonable. I cut back my dosage. I thought that maybe if I just took one per night instead of two, I'd still get enough benefits to move my weight loss from six pounds to seven—it might just take an extra few days. I could live with that. Or maybe if I alternated days . . . yeah, that's what I should do. So I still got the right dose, just not as frequently.

It was only when I started wondering who would find me when my heart gave out, and if it would be in time, that I decided to show myself a little kindness and throw out the pills. Mostly because I didn't want to deal with the paperwork of an emergency room visit—or, worse yet, the call to my parents.

What It Means to Practice Kindness

That small instance of kindness, listening to my body and stopping the pills, didn't feel like much in the moment. In fact, at that time it felt more like throwing in the towel than being kind to myself. But just as my body had been speaking to me for a long time before I noticed it, the same is true of my relationship with kindness—it was calling me long before I knew (or wanted to answer).

But, eventually, answer I did. Not because I wanted to (nothing could have been further from what I wanted at the time), but because after a stark accounting, the results were in. After twenty-plus years, thousands of dollars, and more misery than I care to remember, I still didn't have the body I thought I should. And I certainly wasn't any happier. In reality, each passing year made me less and less happy as I got further and further away from what I thought my body and my life should be.

So through yoga, therapy, journaling, and everything I'd been reading and learning about body acceptance, I (very begrudgingly at first) realized that what I needed wasn't to be harder on myself. I'd done that. On hundreds of "fresh start" Monday mornings. What I needed was to be kinder. After all the resources I'd spent on the opposite approach, I figured it couldn't hurt to try something else for a while and just see what happened.

Practice Kindness in Your Perspective

When I look back on the Overnight Weight Loss pills story and all the stories I've shared with you, sometimes I feel a bit ridiculous. The me of today looks at the me of back then, especially the me who was far from starting her body acceptance journey, and just thinks: "Really?!"

But I try not to get caught up in that perspective. Part of how I treat myself with kindness now is reminding myself that we're all on a journey, and this is mine. My time is much better spent holding love in my heart for past versions of myself than contempt, because each of these stories has been part of my process.

It's possible that you can see that about my story, too. It's usually easier to have grace for someone else than it is for ourselves. So if you're thinking something like this: "Sure, she did some weird stuff, but look where she is today," followed by "I'll never get there" or "body acceptance never works for me" or "I started a diet this morning—what's the point?" I want to take a moment to talk with just you.

I'll give you the bad news first: You're never going to get this practice right. No one is waiting to give you a stamp of approval, and a day isn't coming when you'll never, ever, ever have another negative thought about your body slip into your head, even if only for a second.

But here's the good news: You can't get this practice wrong, either. Outside the need to practice yoga poses in a way that's safe for you, you can't mess it up. You absolutely will have days (weeks, months) when you don't get on your yoga mat at all. Or when you get enticed by a shiny new diet that your sister's dentist's cousin's girlfriend swears by. Or when you feel terrible about your body and wonder why you even bothered with the idea of body acceptance in the first place. All of that *is* going to happen. You can count on it.

But you can also count on this: It's never too late. One way kindness shows up is by looking at the big picture. Remember when we talked earlier about how diets are tricky because they make you think the problem is you, not the flawed system? Well, if you're like me, you may be so entrenched in thinking you're the problem that you forget to look at where else that belief is hiding. And it very well may be hiding in yoga and body acceptance. Days where you don't get on your yoga mat or where you "slip up" and have a closet fit or put your body down aren't signs of failure.

They're signs that you're *in* the process. Because if you weren't, how would you notice the contrast at all? Before you began something like this practice, you didn't notice days you weren't doing yoga because you weren't practicing at all. And you didn't notice times when you were being hard on your body because that's just how you were with your body. There was nothing unusual to notice.

So when you notice these moments of contrast, celebrate! I'm being completely serious. Those moments of noticing are what this whole thing is all about! We all leave ourselves, usually multiple times per day (or per minute if you're me). That's not so much the problem because that's just life. The problem arises when we never come back. And a moment of contrast is an opportunity to come back.

I encourage you to take each time you notice these contrasts as a chance to show yourself kindness. Because you have a big choice here. You can choose to follow your old pattern and follow those negative thoughts further down the hole. Or you can choose your new pattern and, simply by noticing, make a different choice. Very often, you may choose the old first, and even then it's still not too late—because whenever you realize and want another way (even if it's been weeks, months, or longer), you can still come back to your body and yourself.

Choosing the old way is called being human. But each time you choose the new way, you're building a little more resilience to do it again.

Which is exactly what we're looking for.

Practice Kindness with Your Time Line

As you're getting started or going deeper with this process, you will invariably consider how to make yoga more a part of your life. One of my favorite questions from new students is how often they should be practicing yoga. It's one of those opportunities to foreground kindness, even though we rarely think of it that way. Sometimes the students approach this question with enthusiasm: "I'm excited to be here! How often should I try to practice? Every day?" Other times, they approach it with trepidation: "I'm new here and not sure how to begin. I signed up a month ago but haven't started yet. What's wrong with me?"

Regardless of how they present the question, my answer is always the same: "Welcome! My best advice on how to start and sustain a yoga practice is to keep it very simple." The details of when and how often you practice are a *very* tempting place to fall into your old patterns of buckling down on yourself with a Brand-New You Plan. I highly encourage you to resist this temptation as strongly as you can. Why? Because I've seen this stop people from going further in yoga time and time and time again.

And it's completely unnecessary.

No one cares how often or how long you practice yoga. People are way too involved in their own lives to notice. And if you do encounter someone who has an opinion about it, feel free to thank her for her feedback and move on. Your yoga practice is about *you*. It's your space to do what works for you, and that's going to shift and change over time, so even if you do make a plan that works for you now, it's going to change at some point. It's inevitable!

Here's why I don't recommend committing to three times a week, thirty minutes per session, and writing it down on your calendar so you won't skip it: I've done all those things. And even if it's on my calendar, I'll still skip it if I have a pressing reason to—like catching up on the latest episode of a show I'm watching.

Structured plans for getting into any form of movement are everywhere. There's something so appealing about them, much like the appeal of a diet. You get to forget about listening to your body and just follow what someone else (who's usually deemed an expert, therefore someone who knows more than you do) tells you to do. It feels so good to check off the boxes of the days you practiced! To log the data from whatever personal body monitor you may use! To get the satisfaction of being an A+ student!

That is, until you miss a day. And you *know* that's going to happen. Whether that's in six days or six months, it's going to happen. And when it does, because you've set yourself up in a success/failure paradigm, anything that isn't sticking to the program is viewed as a failure. Even though, of course you're going to miss a day. You're human! And humans sometimes miss a day. There's nothing wrong or broken about you when that happens. What's broken is the idea that anyone can stick to the same schedule, day in and day out, and that when he invariably doesn't, he's a failure. Life doesn't give us the same time and energy every day, and we all know the unexpected happens.

But our inner critics, those voices inside that tell us we're not good enough, don't remember that. And sometimes our outer critics don't, either, even if the outer critic is just the chiding tone from the book or website you were reading where you got whatever particular plan you were following in the first place.

As I mentioned, I recommend that you start simply—more simply even than you may be comfortable with. Why? Because when you start simply, it is much easier to keep going. After all, do you usually feel more encouraged when someone is kind to you or when she berates you? Most likely, the answer is you do better when she's kind, and the same is true when you're the one encouraging yourself. So try something like one deep breath per day for a few days and see how it goes. It may feel impossible not to do more than that, and if you do, that's okay, but let your focus be on keeping it very, very simple.

When you show up for your simple practice, it's much easier to get a sense of how it's working for you than when you show up for a complicated practice. You know what I mean, right? Or maybe I'm the only one who has committed to ninety minutes of yoga every day with great enthusiasm—only to burn out 2.3 days later. When you start simply, you will quickly notice—ah, this is perfect. Or, twenty minutes per day isn't doable right now, but ten is great. Or, I'd like to spend a little more time with this. Doing even a two-week experiment with simplicity sets the stage for an attitude of adaptability, which is absolutely what you need to sustain a practice over the long term.

The key here is to let your body be your guide. But if you're new to yoga or knowing what your body wants or needs, that can sometimes feel confusing or impossible. That's why I suggest starting with something like one deep breath or one pose or five minutes or whatever feels almost absurdly doable. Because when your practice is something that doable, it's more likely that you'll do it regularly. And doing your practice regularly is what helps you build the skill of knowing what your body wants and needs. Because when you know that, you'll know what your practice needs to be from day to day and you can roll with it with more ease. And, of course, you'll also better reap all the physical, emotional, and mental benefits of yoga because, you know, you'll actually be doing it rather than skulking in the corner of your own mind, beating yourself up for not sticking with a plan that wasn't aligned to your actual life in the first place.

If you're reading this as a long-time practitioner of yoga who struggles with creating a regular practice, I encourage you to try this, too. Because I know lots of people who have been practicing for a long time, including myself, and it's still a challenge to get on the mat sometimes because, as time passes, things change and you may not be able to practice the way you used to. Too many of us cling to how we used to do things, whether that's how much time we used to have or poses we used to be able to do, and that prevents us from moving forward. It's useful to have times where you try something different with your practice, and this could be the way into something that actually works for the life you have right now.

Now, none of this means you *can't* do more or that doing more is wrong. Of course not; that would be silly. I think of simplicity as a way to start with the end in mind. If you want a regular yoga practice, start in a way that is regular that you can sustain. It's much easier to practice regularly once you have the habit than it is to start from scratch after burning out yet again.

Practice Kindness When You Feel Discouraged

I take the long-term view of my yoga and body acceptance practices. I very much see both practices as something that will be part of the rest of my life. So when I look at it that way, it makes sense to me that it will naturally ebb and flow because that's how life goes. Life is not the same level of busyness or intensity at all times. Some periods of life lend themselves to more time for practice while other periods of life lend themselves to less time for practice. What I think matters the most is that regularity we were just talking about—letting what that means change and grow as needed.

My very favorite tip relating to this is a mind-set shift. For *so many* years I couldn't get into a groove with my yoga practice because I kept trying to force it (that is, myself) to be something that didn't work for me. What I thought I *should* be doing was ninety minutes of practice a day, every day, without fail. But what actually happened is I'd do that for 3.7 days, skip a day or not do a full ninety minutes, do it for 1.3 more days, skip a day, and then give up entirely, so disgusted was I with my inability to do what I thought I should.

After repeating this pattern for over a decade, though, one day I had this little thought: "What *could* my yoga practice be today?" And that was the moment everything changed for me. I don't really believe in moments where the heavens part and angels sing, but if I've ever had one, this might have been it. For *so long* I'd been focused on the *should*s of my practice (that I invented, by the way; no one was forcing me to try to meet those standards), eroding my self-trust each time I didn't follow through.

So when I asked myself what my practice *could* be, I felt nothing but freedom. Because there's always something I *could* do, even if it's taking one deep breath, or checking in with my body and moving how it wants to move for a few minutes in my desk chair, or getting on my mat for a thirty-minute practice of my choosing. In the realm of *could*, it's all possible. I'm able to show up for my practice with what I found to be shocking regularity because *could* allows me to shape my practice to my ever-changing life, not the other way around.

And this is exactly what we've been talking about all along: using yoga, body acceptance, and kindness to set yourself free. Because what matters more in life than having the inner freedom to enjoy it?

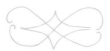

CURVY YOGA

PRACTICES

It's so important to have practices that remind you that kindness toward yourself and your body are possible. Without them, I don't know how it's possible to keep going because there are just too many messages in this world telling us just the opposite.

Practice On and Off the Yoga Mat

We talked about how to make practice part of your life. So here I want to answer some FAQs about practice in case any similar questions might be cooking in your mind.

* What if I skip a day (week, month, year)? Oh, well! I don't mean to be flippant, but I encourage you to take a similarly lighthearted attitude. If you approach your practice in the way we've discussed in this book—a slow and gentle integration into your life—you will find your way forward. As you do, you'll notice that sometimes you skip a day (or however long), or it feels like you do, but when you reflect back you realize you might have been practicing off the mat but not letting it "count." This is not a problem; this is being in the rhythm of your life, with times that lend themselves to more on-the-mat practice and other times to more off-the-mat practice. Moments with more time to practice and others with less. Times with more intensity and others with less. The longer

you practice, the more you see and make peace with your own natural ebb and flow. You can't fail at this because at its core, this practice is your life. It is the answer to the question: "What if it isn't possible to burn out or fail?"

* What if I can't physically practice yoga? Of course, you should always consult and follow your doctor's advice regarding what is best for your body. But I believe there's almost always a way for any and every body to practice yoga. The difference is that it might not always be what you think it "should" be. Remember that shift from *should* to *could*, though? That's perfect in this situation. Could you take one deep breath? Could you stretch your arms overhead, or do some neck stretches, or apply the practice in your everyday life? Open up your ideas about what the practice can be and see if you don't find some ways in. On the physical practice of yoga, you might consider private yoga sessions, seeing a yoga therapist, taking classes from someone specialized in an area where your body needs support, or something along those lines.

* What if I'm still critical of my body sometimes? Oh my goodness, welcome to the club! I truly do not know one person who doesn't have these thoughts pop up from time to time, even if very few and far between. In my own life, I treat those critical moments as opportunities to do the practice—presence, get curious, challenge, and affirm. I'm actually almost happy to have those moments now, not because I love having the thoughts, but because I've noticed them. Noticing them gives me the opportunity to do the practice and start to make a shift. With noticing, I at least have a chance, unlike the days when I didn't even notice the thoughts because they were so pervasive. Also, I've benefitted greatly from the support of professionals such as psychotherapists, yoga teachers, life coaches, body-positive doctors, and nutritionists.

 What if I go on another diet? I hate to be a broken record here, but again—oh, well. You've likely inscribed that pattern for many, many years. It makes sense you might find yourself there again. I can't even tell you how many times I perused new diets, tried them for a while, backed away, and repeated the cycle when I was at the beginning (and not-so-beginning) stages of my body acceptance journey. It's all part of it. You've been trained for years to put your focus in one place (weight) and how you're shifting your focus to another (the behaviors that support you physically, mentally, and emotionally, independent of your weight). Sometimes you might not even notice you're on a diet for a while! That's okay, too. Do your practice again and see what arises.

 What if people in my life think accepting your body is a bad idea? I'm sorry to say this is not uncommon. The people in our lives, just like us, are living in a system where thin is equated with status and health. It can be very challenging for people in our lives to see us choose a different way, particularly if they're still holding themselves to the standards of that system. I recommend finding a go-to phrase you can use to exit those conversations if you don't want to get into it, something like "I know it might not be what you're used to, but I'm trying it." Or "Thank you for your input, but I don't want to discuss this." And, of course, if you want to tell them more, you totally can! The main thing I suggest is doing whatever best supports you staying centered in your body and being.

Body Gratitude

Another wonderful way to connect with and show appreciation for your body is through a body gratitude meditation. This can take a couple of forms, which can work together or separately, depending on what you need.

As usual, begin in a comfortable position, and then:

* Turn your attention to your feet. Make any movements with your feet that feel good for you. When you've completed that, allow your feet to relax and grow still. Now, think of one simple thing you can thank your feet for. Once you have stated that gratitude to yourself, continue up the body from there, moving to your legs, hips, belly, back, hands, arms, shoulders, neck, and head.

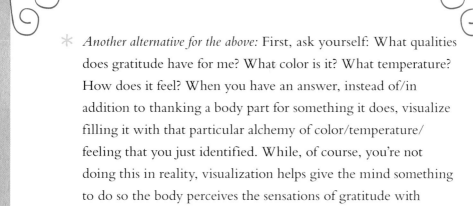

✳ *Another alternative for the above:* First, ask yourself: What qualities does gratitude have for me? What color is it? What temperature? How does it feel? When you have an answer, instead of/in addition to thanking a body part for something it does, visualize filling it with that particular alchemy of color/temperature/feeling that you just identified. While, of course, you're not doing this in reality, visualization helps give the mind something to do so the body perceives the sensations of gratitude with greater ease and clarity. Continue this process until your whole body is filled with the color/temperature/feeling of gratitude.

You may feel complete with this process once you finish one of the options above. However, if you'd like to deepen your body gratitude even more or try something different next time, here's an option:

✳ Visualize in front of you someone or something that it's easy for you to feel abundant gratitude for. Don't make it someone you have a complicated relationship with. Make it simple: a beloved pet, your favorite person on earth, a glorious tree. It doesn't matter who or what it is, as long as you can easily feel a great amount of gratitude for them/it.

✳ Once you have visualized that, visualize your own heart, then add in a visualization of a ribbon connecting your heart to the person/thing in front of you. Once that is established, ask yourself: Where in my body do I feel gratitude for this person/thing? It might be right there at your heart, and/or it may be somewhere else, which could be an expected or unexpected location.

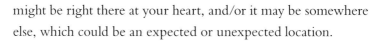

* Now, ask yourself: How could I magnify, or intensify, this feeling of gratitude? Do I need to lengthen my spine? Breathe more deeply? Relax my forehead? When you have an answer, carry out that action.

* Fold your hands in front of your heart and bow to the person/object in front of you, thanking that person/object for its presence in your life. Then gently reel that ribbon of connection back into your heart, knowing you can reconnect with that person/object anytime in the future.

* Next, visualize yourself in front of you. Begin the process from above: Visualize a ribbon connecting your actual heart to the heart of the you in front of you. Return to the location of gratitude in your body that you'd just found, and extend that gratitude to yourself. Take the earlier action to nurture that feeling of gratitude even more.

* When you feel complete with that, instead of just inviting the ribbon back within, this time invite yourself and the ribbon into your heart. After all, you were there all along; sometimes we just need a reminder.

Internal/External Integration

If you've ever felt disconnected from your body, and particularly if you've often felt that way throughout your life, it can be challenging to have a sense of your own wholeness, particularly in the world at large. That's why I love this last practice so much. It can be a profound reminder that not only are you inherently whole, but that you can maintain that sense as you go about your everyday life, too. It really is the culmination of the process I've laid out in this book. To try this:

* Begin in a comfortable, lying-down (or seated) position.

* Notice where you are in contact with whatever you are sitting/ lying on. What are the differences in your body side to side? Where do you feel warmth or coolness? What adjustments could you make to your position to be more comfortable?

* Once you are settled in, turn next to hearing. What's the first thing you hear? Once you've noticed that, listen underneath: What else is present for you to hear that you may not have noticed at first?

* Now, do the same with smell. What's the first smell you pick up? And what about the second?

* Then, do the same with sight, even if your eyes are closed. What colors and patterns of light/shadow do you pick up, even behind your eyelids? What else do you see once you notice what first presents itself for your attention?

* Finally, do the same with taste. What tastes do you pick up in your mouth? What is the difference front to back, side to side?

* Once you have engaged all five senses, expand your awareness through your whole body and sense outward, getting a sense of yourself on whatever you're sitting/lying on, then in the room, then in the building, then in the neighborhood, then in the town.

* When you have a sense of where you are in space, redirect that attention inward and ask yourself: What can I notice here? If I could describe my feeling state in one word, what would it be? Where do I feel movement happening within, perhaps from my breath or the beating of my heart?

* When you have a sense of your inner experience, expand your awareness through your whole body, inviting in all of yourself.

* Finally, from this sense of inner wholeness, notice yourself again in space, knowing that you can always maintain this external sensing (perception) with internal sensing (interoception) in a state of integration.

As your journey continues, I encourage you to return to the practices throughout this book that you find most help you connect with yourself. It's powerful to see how your experience of them changes over time; they can each act as their own Barometer for the practice that is getting to know, accept, and maybe even love your body and yourself.

IT'S NOT
possible
TO LOVE
yourself
TOO MUCH.
Keep going!

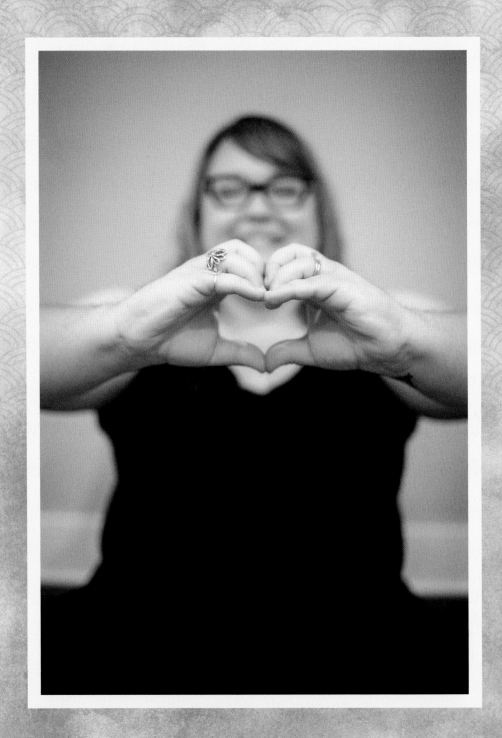

Afterword

My husband and I went on a vacation to the Pacific Northwest not too long ago. We were mostly out in remote areas with no cell service, which was such a refreshing change of pace.

In the past when we've been on vacation, it's taken me several days to unwind enough to truly relax. It usually wasn't until the last day that I'd feel my jaw unclench, that I could go with the flow and not be controlling about our plan for the day, or that I wouldn't spend the majority of my time avoiding being seen in my bathing suit or finding reasons not to go for a walk because I hadn't moved my body for fun in so long that I didn't know what it would be like. Once I began to finally loosen up on things, I'd spend the rest of the trip mourning how it had taken me so long to do so and fearing how long it would be until I got to feel this good again.

This time, though, things were different. Around the second day, I noticed that I was already going with the flow, sleeping well, happy to traipse around wherever. And because it was so strange to me, my first thought wasn't "How great!" Instead, it was "Am I doing this vacation right? How am I already so relaxed? What am I missing here?"

And then it hit me: I was already relaxed because I had so much inner ease in my overall life. I didn't have as far to come down on vacation as I had in the past, so I was free to just enjoy it.

When I had that insight, I smiled and proceeded to do just that. We spent the rest of the trip marveling at the beauty of where we were, going for lots of hikes, sleeping in, letting the day take us where it would, and just generally being happy to have time away and with each other.

During this trip, I didn't obsess about my body—in a bad way or a good way. I wasn't concerned with how many calories I consumed or didn't consume at dinner, and I didn't log my steps on our hikes as a way to secretly congratulate myself. In addition, I also didn't spend any time running through fields exclaiming how much I love and am grateful for my body.

I simply lived, free from body hatred and free to soak up the sun, the rest, the beauty.

This is what I'd wanted all those years and thought I'd get from dieting but never did (because it doesn't reside there): the ability to live life on my own terms and feel it all, absorbing the fullness of this always-short human life that is mine and mine alone.

Looking Back and Forward

To say that I'm grateful to have not had an experience like the one with the Overnight Weight Loss pills in years is an understatement of dramatic proportions. Though I can still imagine being fleetingly tempted by something like that more as a conditioned response than anything else, I can no longer imagine even seriously considering buying them, much less actually taking them.

The reason isn't that I had one great epiphany and changed my life. It's more like I had 100,000 small insights, forgot most of them, and implemented a few in fits and starts (mostly fits). There's definitely no "Overnight Body Acceptance" pill.

Though that might be one I'd be more tempted to take.

There are always new layers to uncover in this process, such as when I recently injured my left achilles tendon and wasn't able to hike or practice much yoga for a bit. I found myself being so hard on myself, feeling that if only I'd had a different body, that never would have happened. But, of course, bodies get injured, no matter what their shape or size. And whether through injury, illness, aging, or some other change, there are always new components of this practice to work with—or revisit.

Was I not living and enjoying life sometimes when I was obsessed with my body, onto my next diet, caught in a seemingly unending shame spiral? Of course I was—at least some of the time. But my mind was so distracted by all those other preoccupations that very often I didn't recognize it, much less remember it. I missed out on so many sweet experiences, conversations with friends and family, and time with myself by letting that inner critic in my head take control, giving far more attention to wondering if my friend was horrified by how I looked than listening carefully to what she had to say.

Before I started this journey, I spent so much time thinking *about* my body, and almost no time living *in* and enjoying and appreciating my body. The beauty of what this practice has brought to my life is that now those two are nearly reversed. Now, I spend much more time just living my life, moving and checking in with my body, and much less time thinking *about* it (especially all the things I don't like about it, which used to occupy at least 95 percent of my brain at any given moment).

This is what I want for you, too. I want you to know in your bones that your body is worthy of your love right now. No exceptions. I want yoga to be a support and friend for you, a way to stay connected with yourself— especially when it feels impossible. I want you to free up your time, resources, mental energy, emotions, and anything else you have invested in hating your body and channel those into living and loving your life. As far as I know, this may be the only one we get—so let's live it out to its edges, not measured out in half-cup and pound by pound increments.

Next Steps in Your Practice

As you move forward from here, remember that this is a new landscape. It isn't what may be the familiar feeling of outsourcing your relationship with your body—of letting diet books, health "experts," your cousin, or your partner tell you what you should or shouldn't do. Instead, it's the shoes-off, feet-in-the-dirt practice of feeling and noticing. Forgetting and remembering. Leaving yourself and coming back. It doesn't matter how long it takes you to come back, or how terrible you felt while you were away. All that matters is picking yourself up, not even beginning again, because coming back isn't starting over. It's a continuation of a long conversation with yourself.

The beginning of a yoga practice is mostly about figuring out where to put your feet and arms, and how to stay in alignment, and maybe how to breathe. This makes sense; it's how we all are with something new. But once you have a better sense of how to move in your body, that doesn't have to be the sole focus.

You can invite in *more* feeling.

So next time you're on your mat, engage in the practice:

* Where is my body right now? What am I in contact with?

* What is happening in X part of my body? Or with my breath?

* If negative or doubtful thoughts are arising, how can I challenge them?

* Then let yourself be, affirming your body.

When you allow this practice to guide you, it will take you where you're meant to go next on your path. After all, yoga isn't about getting better at yoga poses. Nor is body acceptance about getting better at body acceptance.

Both are about living your life. And you can work with that process no matter what yoga pose you can or can't do physically.

Hear Me

Here's the truth that I hope you feel calling you through the beating of your own heart, no matter how far away the sound may seem in this moment: No one knows your own body better than you do. So when you hear something on TV about the latest diet/health trend, or read something about it in a magazine, or get caught listening to the details of what your neighbor is doing with it, hold it all gently.

Start by noticing when your body may be sending you messages. Is this something that feels right to and for you? Do you find yourself going into hyperplanning mode, visualizing how perfect your life will be once you implement that plan exactly? Be on the lookout for times when that fantasy life presents itself, and get curious. Also, look underneath—what is it that you *truly* want from that "ideal" body? Is it more happiness or freedom, greater ease in your body? If so, see what you can do to start bringing those things into your life *now*. Pay attention to how you feel. Focus on bringing in more good and making your life fuller, not smaller. If you have questions, look for a body-affirming health professional or yoga teacher to consult.

As you go along with that, challenge whatever assumptions come up, because they always do. You will run into many things that tell you that you can't be trusted, that your body can't be trusted. When you do, take those as another opportunity to check in and ask yourself: "Is that true?" And "What if my body isn't a problem?"

If you're feeling stuck and unsure of which way to turn, let yoga be your companion in tuning in to yourself, however often you remember and need to do that. Yoga isn't yet another thing to feel bad about—how you do it, not doing it enough, or whatever other strictures we like to set up for ourselves.

As your journey and life continue to unfold, keep kindness front and center, and keep coming back to your body again and again and again, affirming it.

What I really want you to know is that this practice is yours to make of it what you will. There's no prescription here. There's just practice, working its way down deep into your bones. This isn't a lifestyle, but a way to be alive. It's not a fix-yourself plan; it's a know-and-support-yourself invitation.

I hope you carry this practice onto your yoga mat and let it grow from there into the rest of your life.

Make it yours.

I can't wait to hear where it takes you.

Curvy Loving-Kindness Meditation

I'm going to close this book the same way I close many of my yoga classes: with a loving-kindness meditation I wrote. You're welcome to use this meditation any time you want, as often as you want. (And you can grab a recording of it on my website if you'd like.)

Take a deep breath to begin, then repeat these phrases to yourself:

May I greet my body with gentleness.

May I soften when life invites me to harden.

May I listen to my intuition with wisdom and trust it with ease.

May I appreciate my body a little more in this moment, just as it is.

The light in me honors the light in you.

YOGA
leads the way
TO
body acceptance
BY CONNECTING
you to you

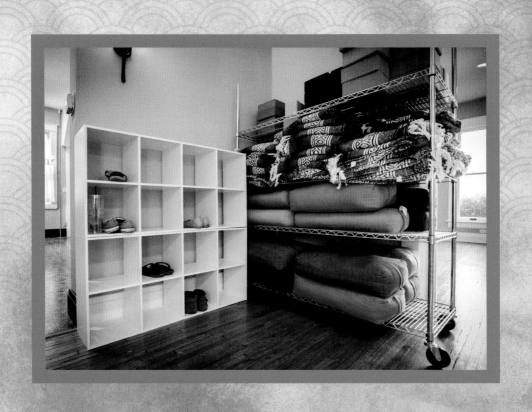

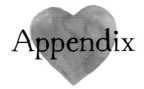

Appendix

Yoga Poses Should Work for You

Not the Other Way Around

When I think back on all the years I spent practicing yoga, hoping no one would notice how, when the teacher suggested that we "place our bellies on our thighs," I only had to move a centimeter to get there, I cringe a little. Not for the reason I would have thought, which is being embarrassed by my body, but because I could have been so much more comfortable—if only I'd known a few simple things!

What I want for you is to know how to make yoga poses work for your body so that you can practice with more comfort, safety, stability, and ease right now—whether you're brand-new to yoga or have been practicing for years and are ready to make things work for you a bit better.

If you want to practice in a Curvy Yoga class, you have several options, including finding a certified teacher near you and joining our virtual studio.[1]

In addition to those choices, you can also use Curvy Yoga principles in any classes you attend or in your home practice.

The following pose instructions and options are intended to support you in crafting a yoga practice to fit your own needs. This way, whether on your own or in any type of class, you'll always know that you can make the poses work for you. I've focused the instructions here on curvy-specific pose options, as well as a few key poses seen in yoga classes, so that you can apply the information to any style of yoga you may practice. I've listed the poses by their common English names, as well as their Sanskrit names. Many pose names differ across various styles of yoga, though, so the principles I'm describing are relevant to the movement and action of the pose, regardless of the name.

Because of the wide range of yoga poses that exist, I have not attempted to describe every pose possible. Instead, I've focused on key poses, where curvy principles are readily available, so that you can apply those principles to other similar poses you may encounter.

As with any form of movement, be sure to consult a doctor before beginning the practice to make sure you are able to participate and to know how to do so safely. If you feel pain when engaging in any form of movement, stop immediately and consult a doctor before proceeding.

Props

Yoga props are tools that help you make yoga poses work for you. Yoga props (blocks, blanket, bolster, strap, chair, and more) allow you to work through the pose in a way that makes sense for your body. They offer relief and release, support and stability.

Just as support from a loved one or a colleague can make all the difference sometimes, yoga props help you find your version of the pose. And if you think that doesn't matter all that much, consider that if you can't make the pose work for you, you may well feel discouraged and that yoga isn't for you. But yoga is for you; you just have to find out what you need to make it so. And there's nothing like a well-placed yoga prop, with some clear instructions on how to use it, to make that happen.

The goal of props isn't to get rid of them. Though you may eventually dial the blocks under your hands in a Standing Forward Bend down from the high to the medium height, you may or may not ever get rid of them entirely. The goal isn't to get rid of them—or to keep them. The goal is to use them as appropriate for your body today. Because if the only goal is to get rid of them, on the day you need them again (which will inevitably happen at some point—tightness after a long day of travel, injury/illness, just being tired), you may feel as if you've done something wrong. But if you see the props as something to always check in with to assess where you are that day, it's not possible to get it wrong (and it never was in the first place; it just doesn't always feel that way).

For the following pose options, you might like to have these yoga props, or supports, available. You will not need every prop for every pose, and you might not need some of these at all, but I still want to introduce them to you so you're familiar with them. While the actual props are great, you can also use household equivalents, so I'll explain both choices for all the props I describe.

Yoga mat There are many different types and sizes of mats available, and I think what you choose is a matter of personal preference. If you are starting from square one and don't have a mat, I recommend considering one of the thicker varieties (somewhere around ¼" thick). I find that they provide better cushioning for joints.
Household equivalent If you do not have a yoga mat, you may be able to practice without one on the flooring that you have. One function of a mat is to provide stability, so as long as your floor isn't slippery, you may be fine without one. Another function of a mat is to provide some cushioning, so if you have noncarpeted floors, you might want to put a rug down on the floor, as long as that doesn't cause the floor to become slippery. If you have carpeted floors, it just depends on the pile of the carpet. Some carpeted floors will be stable and comfortable for you; others might not be.

Two yoga blocks Yoga blocks are relatively easy to find these days; you can often find them in general-type stores, and you can also find them online. I recommend four-inch (10-cm) foam blocks, though they come in different sizes and materials (if you already have some of a different kind, just go with what you have). Yoga blocks have three heights: high, medium, and low. The purpose of these blocks is to bring the floor to you (e.g., underneath your hands in a Standing Forward Bend if your hands don't reach the floor), so start with the most accessible height of the block (it depends on what you're doing as to what that will be) and then decrease the support if you find that's warranted, which usually means you can maintain alignment and stability without strain with the lessened support. I like having two blocks when possible (one under each hand in something like Standing Forward Bend), but one will suffice.

Household equivalent Because a major purpose of blocks is to bring the floor to you, you can use almost any stable thing you have around, including a couple of dense books, a coffee table (if you're just putting your hands on it in a Standing Forward Bend, for example, not if you're bearing weight), a couple of canned goods, and the like. The possibilities are many; just make sure you choose something stable for the purpose you intend to use it for.

Yoga strap The purpose of a strap (also sometimes called a yoga belt) is to extend the reach of your arms. Straps are also relatively easy to find; they're usually next to yoga blocks in stores, or you can find them online. I recommend a ten-foot (3-m) strap. The ten-foot (3-m) strap is longer than many you'll see, but I think it's great because it gives you a little more space to do whatever you may want.

Household equivalent To get the ten-foot (3-m) length, you may need to find some rope or something like that. If you don't have that, though, it's totally fine to use something of a shorter length because that will work for almost all occasions. An old necktie, a scarf, a cloth belt from a robe, or other things like that work perfectly!

Sturdy chair The yoga and household equivalents are the same here: a stable chair without wheels.

Yoga blanket Yoga blankets have a density to them that can provide nice support as well as cushioning. These may be harder to find in a local store (though certainly not impossible!) but are easily available online. **Household equivalent** This is one prop that's very easy to find a household equivalent for. You can use any dense blanket you may have. Towels, particularly beach towels, also work well.

One yoga bolster Bolsters are similar to very firm pillows and come in both round and rectangular sizes. I use a rectangular bolster because I find it to be somewhat more versatile, but if you already have a round one, that will be fine for most things, too.
Household equivalent A firm pillow will work well for most bolster purposes. When looking around your house for one, don't forget pillows you may have on a couch/bed for decoration and/or couch cushions as options. If you don't have anything that will work pillow-wise, a tightly rolled-up firm blanket or towel (beach towels can be nice) will also work for most occasions.

Wall space I offer some options in this book for using a wall for support. It will be nice if you can practice where you can bring the short end of your mat up against a wall and not risk knocking anything off.

Now let's get to the poses! For each pose you'll find some different options to experiment with. My hope here is that you can see what works for you and doesn't, so bring that attitude of curiosity we talked about earlier with you, and we'll get into it.

Easy Seat | *Sukhasana*

Come to a sitting position on the floor. I recommend that you sit on a folded-up blanket or something of similar density to lift your hips up. Doing so gives a bit more freedom to the hips, which in turn gives more space for the rest of the body to settle in more comfortably. If you do sit on a blanket, try sitting more toward the front of it. This can help your pelvis come into a more neutral position, particularly if you're not used to sitting on the floor (which is true for many of us!).

Cross your legs in front of you, crossing at the shins or ankles, whichever is possible for you. Once you've done this, lean a little to the left and place your right hand under your right hip/bum. Lightly hold the skin of the hip/bum and move it out to the right a bit and back. This allows you to get more onto your sitz bones (the bones you're sitting on), which provides grounding for this position. Repeat on the other side.

Next option: If you feel like you can't get a comfy seat yet and/or your thighs feel compressed, bring your right hand to the inside of your left inner thigh. Bring your left hand to the outside of your left thigh so you are holding your thigh between your hands. Using your hands, roll the thigh skin down and under (to the left). Repeat on the other side. This can also help you get grounded, in addition to giving your legs a little more room.

Another choice: If your belly feels compressed, lean your torso back a bit. Bring your left hand to the bottom of the left side of your belly (near where your torso meets your hip). Do the same on the right side. With your hands on either side of your belly, take hold of the belly and move it down toward your pelvis. Bring your torso back to center. This action can make your belly rest more comfortably. If that doesn't work for your body, you can also do the reverse: Bring your hands to the same place but this time lift the belly skin up, placing it back down once you're settled.

After you make these adjustments, if the knees are higher than the hips, support them in one of a couple of ways. (1) Sit up on more height until the

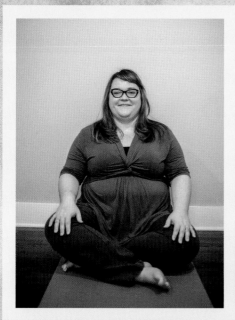
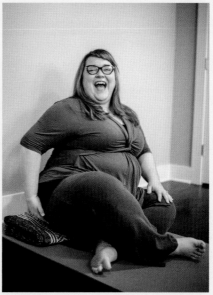

knees can begin to drop down. This may mean sitting on two blankets, a bolster, or whatever you have on hand until you find a height that works for you. (2) Place a block or another support under each knee so that the knees can rest into the blocks for support. If the highest height of the block feels best for you but also feels like it may fall over, you can stack two blocks on the low height instead, if you have them available.

Application to other poses: You can make these or similar adjustments to other seated poses, particularly cross-legged ones. You can also do the bum and belly adjustments when seated in a chair if sitting on the floor doesn't work for you.

Cat/Cow | *Chakravakasana*

This pose is traditionally done from hands and knees, but I'm going to offer you a seated version first. This seated version is great if kneeling isn't an option for you; it can be done from the floor, a chair, or just about anywhere! It's also nice for helping to feel the actions of the spine in this pose before trying it from hands and knees if you're able to do that.

Seated

Begin in Easy Seat as before. If you're seated in a chair, sit in such a way that you can bring your feet to the floor, if possible. If not, sit so that you can lengthen your spine.

With your hands on your legs, inhale and lift your sternum (or breastbone), coming into a small back arch. You can lean a bit forward with the torso as you do this, keeping your head in line with your spine (meaning you don't drop your head back).

Then, exhale and lightly tuck your chin to your chest as you round your back and lean back. The hands on the legs can provide some support for this movement, allowing you to round your back more.

Continue like this, moving at the pace of your own breath. Repeat five to ten times.

Kneeling

Come onto your hands and knees, with your hands underneath your shoulders and your knees underneath your hips in a neutral position, often called Tabletop. You might like to have your knees on a blanket or a kneepad here if the mat alone is uncomfortable.

Before you go anywhere, press down under the fleshy root of the thumb on each hand (located in the palm). This can help to relieve pressure in the wrist. Do the same under the root of both index fingers. Additionally, press underneath all of your fingertips.

From here, inhale and reach your sternum forward then up as you also lift

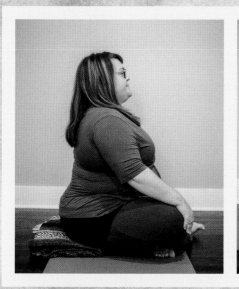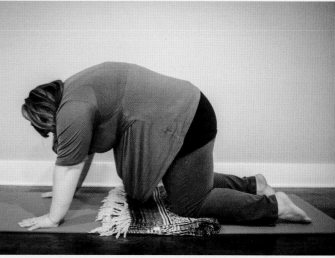

your tailbone up. Doing this will bring your back into a small arch, similar to the seated version. As earlier, from the seated position, keep your head in line with your spine.

Next, exhale and begin to take your spine in the opposite direction: tuck your chin toward your chest and round your back up.

Continue like this, moving at the pace of your own breath. Repeat five to ten times.

Application to other poses: You can use the idea of moving a pose that is traditionally done on the knees to another position for any kneeling poses. For example, you could move Camel (*Ustrasana*) to seated on a chair or Gate (*Parighasana*) to standing with one leg on a chair seat. In addition, adding support underneath the knees can work in any kneeling pose. We talked more about this in Chapter Five.

Mountain | *Tadasana*

The distance between the feet in this pose is what determines your base of support. The goal is to find a base of support that allows you to feel grounded while still stacking hips over knees over ankles to support your joints well.

This pose is sometimes taught with feet together (see Chapter Five for more info on this). In the photo, I am able to stand with my feet together. You may be able to see, though, how that causes my thighs to compress, and therefore my knees roll in. This position is unstable for my body; if someone even brushed past me, I'd topple right over. I also feel squeezed like a tube of toothpaste, unable to take a full breath. It is not a wide-enough base of support for my body, though it may be for yours. That's what the following experiment is for.

Begin standing with your feet as close together as possible and observe how you feel. Are you able to press down firmly underneath the ball of each big toe, underneath the ball of each pinky toe, and underneath the center of each heel? Do you feel rooted and balanced, as though you could stand your ground if someone brushed past you? Do you have space to take a deep breath? If the answer to all these questions is yes, this may be the right position for you.

If the answer to one or more of these questions is no, though, we'll begin to experiment. Step your feet hip distance apart (meaning the internal hip bones; see Chapter Five for more info on this). Review the questions above and assess. If you find you need more space, step the feet another inch (2.5 cm) apart, continuing until you find the position that is right for you. As I mentioned above, stacking hips over knees over ankles is the most supported structural position (as opposed to having the feet much wider than the hips, for example). However, if that is not stable for you, step wider bit by bit until you find the position where you feel steady and not squeezed like a tube of toothpaste but can still stack your joints. For most people who find they need more room, this is just a bit wider than hip distance.

Once you find the appropriate distance between your feet, we can move on to the rest of the position.

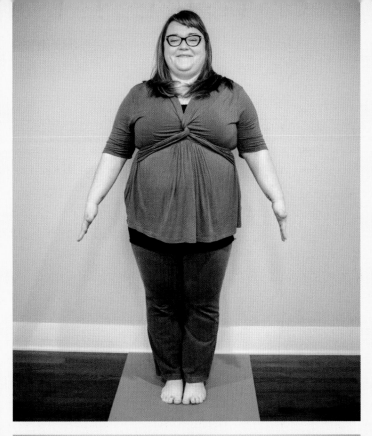

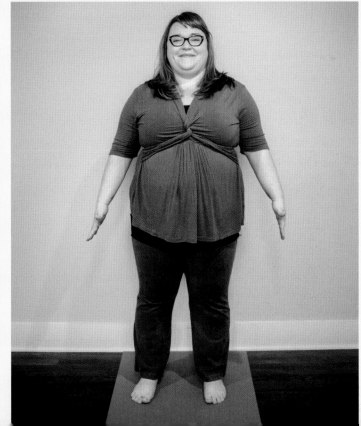

Mountain | *Tadasana* (continued)

Bring a microbend into your knees. A microbend is a bend so small that someone else might not even be able to see it, but you can feel it. The purpose of the microbend in your knees is to prevent your knees from locking.

Hips stay over the knees. You want the pelvis to be in what is sometimes known as a neutral position, meaning that you are neither tucking your tailbone down nor popping it out.

Now, lift your sternum a bit and broaden across your collarbones (meaning, don't allow them to round in). Next, create space between your shoulder blades on your back, finding evenness in the shoulders so they are neither rounding forward nor back.

Arms can be active by the sides with fingertips pointing, or palms can turn to face forward.

Soften the sides of your neck between your ears and shoulders (let your shoulders drop down). Your gaze is looking forward, chin parallel to the ground.

This is a lot of instruction for what we often think of as "just" standing! However, we can learn so much from this pose, including what it feels like to press through the feet and lengthen all the way through the body. This is a feeling and action we will return to—and that you can revisit anytime, anywhere.

Application to other poses: You can use the standing principles, particularly the work of the feet and legs, in many other standing poses because this pose is very often the foundation.

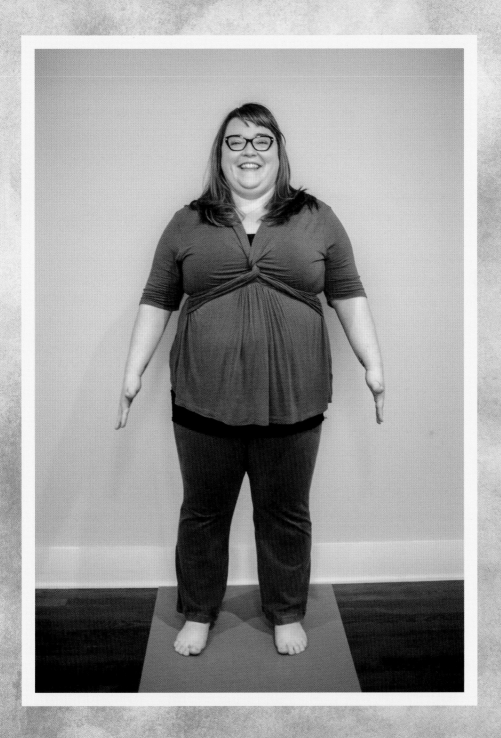

Standing Forward Bend | *Uttanasana*

Begin in Mountain Pose. Lightly draw your navel toward your spine.

Inhale, raising your arms above your head, palms facing each other.

Exhale and bend your knees as you begin to fold forward from the hips, bringing your hands down to two blocks. Let your head release down.

If you do not have blocks or their equivalent available, you can also bring your hands to your thighs, shins, or the floor.

If your belly feels compressed, step your feet a little wider apart (perhaps an inch [2.5 cm] or so) until you get a little more space to release your spine and head down.

Legs are working toward straight (not necessarily *to* straight, just in that general direction). If the legs are straight (but not locked; keep at least a microbend in the knees) and you have your hands on the blocks, check and see if you naturally have space to bend your elbows. If you do, that tells you that you can play with dialing your blocks down to the medium height. You can then repeat that process and perhaps dial the blocks down to the low height or remove them.

If your chest feels like it's strangling/suffocating you or like you can't release your head down, take a moment and lengthen the spine so it's roughly parallel to the floor. Tuck your chin towards your chest here, then release the head down. Your face will be closer to your chest, but there's more space in the neck.

If you'd like even more space for the belly, the next time you try this pose, before you fold forward, bring your hands to either side of your low belly. Press the skin in and down toward the hips as much as possible (without pain; don't push too hard!). As you fold forward, skip raising the arms overhead and just fold forward from here. Once the upper body comes down, you can release your hands from your hips and bring them to the blocks because gravity and your torso will keep the skin where you moved it.

Application to other poses: You can use the technique of tucking the chin before folding all the way forward in other forward bends, including seated, as well as poses like Down Dog.

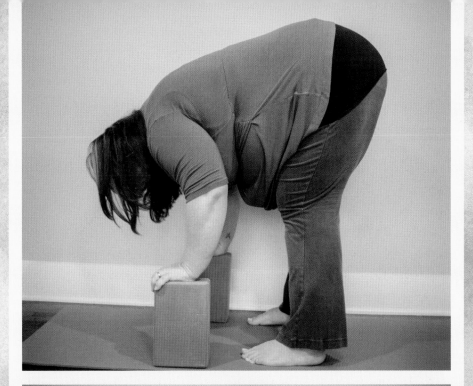

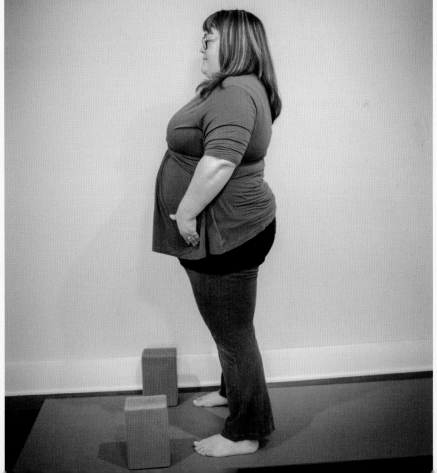

Down Dog | *Adho Mukha Svanasana*

If this pose isn't comfortable or available to you from the floor, try these two great options to access the same areas of the body.

Wall

Begin by facing a wall, approximately arms-distance away.

Press your hands into the wall at the height of your hips. Before you go anywhere, press down under the root of the thumb and first finger on both hands, as well as all ten of your fingertips.

From here, begin walking your feet back with your knees slightly bent, allowing your torso to come forward with your head facing the floor.

Once you've walked back to a point where your spine is roughly parallel to the floor with your arms extended, begin working your legs toward straight. Reach your tailbone toward the wall behind you as you press your thighs back. Your ears should be roughly in line with your biceps.

Take several breaths here.

When you're ready to come out of the pose, bend your knees and slowly walk forward until you can comfortably bring your torso up and come to standing. Once you're standing, gently release your arms from the wall.

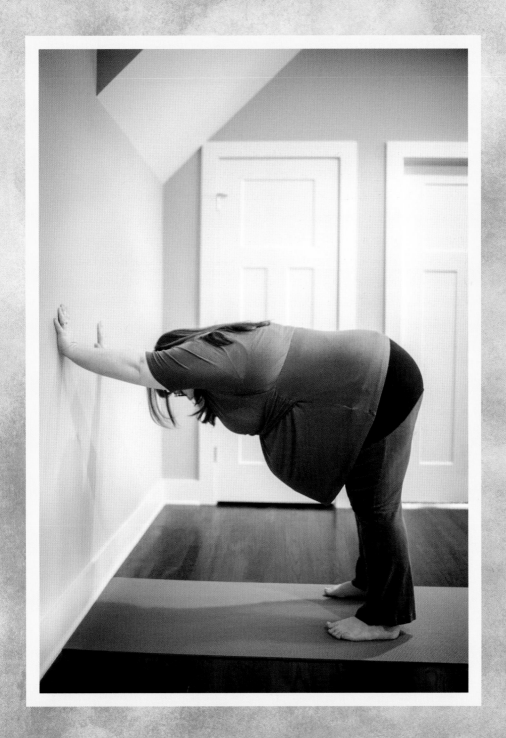

Down Dog | *Adho Mukha Svanasana*
(*continued*)

Chair

The chair version of this pose is very similar to the wall version. The bonus here is that it often allows for even more opening through the backs of the legs and extension through the spine.

Begin by standing facing a chair (with the seat toward you), about half a foot in front of it, in Mountain Pose. It's best if the chair is in front of a wall, with the back legs in contact, so it's stable.

Inhale and reach your arms overhead; exhale and fold forward as in Standing Forward Bend, this time bringing your hands to the chair seat. Press both hands flat into the chair seat and press underneath the hands as in Cat/Cow. If the chair seat is slippery or there's another reason why your hands can't be flat on the chair seat, turn your hands to the side and grip the sides of the chair seat.

Begin to walk your feet back, as in the wall version. The difference here is that the body will make more of a "V" shape with the chair than an "L" shape with the wall.

Again, work the legs toward straight, lengthening through your spine, ears about in line with the biceps. Press your thighs back as you work your legs toward straight.

Take several breaths here.

When you've completed that, walk your feet forward to a Standing Forward Bend with hands still on the chair seat. Then when you feel ready, press through your feet and bring yourself up to standing.

Application to other poses: The wall and chair can be nice supports for other poses.

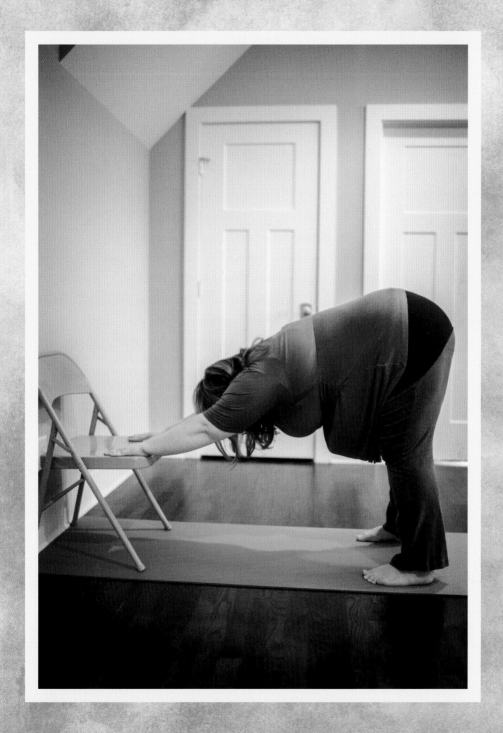

Sun Salutations | *Surya Namaskar*

Sun Salutations, sometimes also called *vinyasas*, are a linked series of poses. While these poses follow a traditional sequence, it's not uncommon for this to be changed up a bit, depending on your class or teacher. In general, though, we can assume a similar sequence of poses.

Oftentimes, the trickiest part of a traditional Sun Salutation for a curvy practitioner is the moment when you step forward from Down Dog to Standing Forward Bend. The reason this is complicated is that the instruction is often given to step one foot directly forward, either behind the hand in front of you or between the hands. If you have anything happening in the belly or chest area, though, as soon as you go to step that foot forward, your knee is going to get stuck on one, the other, or both. This not only feels uncomfortable, it can also get you out of the rhythm of the rest of the class if you're practicing in a group setting. There's no problem with that, of course; I think it's fine to take your time. But sometimes people do feel awkward about it, and there's no reason that has to happen!

Here are my favorite two options for stepping forward from Down Dog while in a Sun Salutation.

One Knee Down

One great option is to bring the opposite knee down. For example, if you're stepping the right foot forward, you would bring the left knee gently to the ground. The knee on the ground will give you some support and stability for making space for the right leg to come forward.

Once the left knee is down, shift a little to your left until the right leg can get free. Step the right leg a bit wide, bringing it behind and/or outside the right hand. I say "a bit wide" because it's impossible to give an exact measurement that would suit everyone. You're not swinging the leg out as far to the right as it can go; you're just stepping it about an inch or so (2–5 cm) to the right so you have enough space to come forward. When the front foot is securely forward, shift yourself back to center, tuck your left toes under, engage your

(continued)

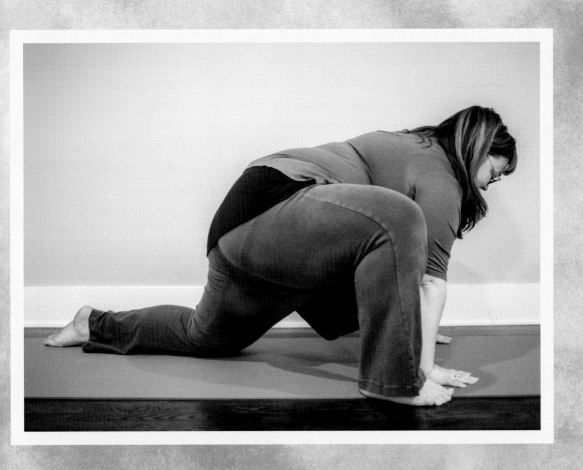

core and lift your hips up. Finally, lean back a little with your hips and then use that action to get a little help stepping your left foot forward in one or more steps. Once both feet are up, step the feet closer together before coming up.

Stepping Wide

Sometimes you may not be able to bring your knee down to the ground comfortably and/or you may not feel you have time to do so. In that case, another option is simply to step wide.

From Down Dog, shift slightly to your left as you step the right leg forward and wide, in one or more steps. Again, we are talking about stepping the foot an inch or so (2–5 cm) wide. From there, bring your left foot forward in one or more steps as described in the one-knee-down option.

Another choice for stepping wide is to step both feet wide and walk the feet up one at a time until you come to the front, then step the feet back closer together for your Standing Forward Bend. Alternately, you could walk the hands to the feet.

Application to other poses: You can use the wide step anytime you are stepping forward, whether from a pose like Down Dog or a High Lunge.

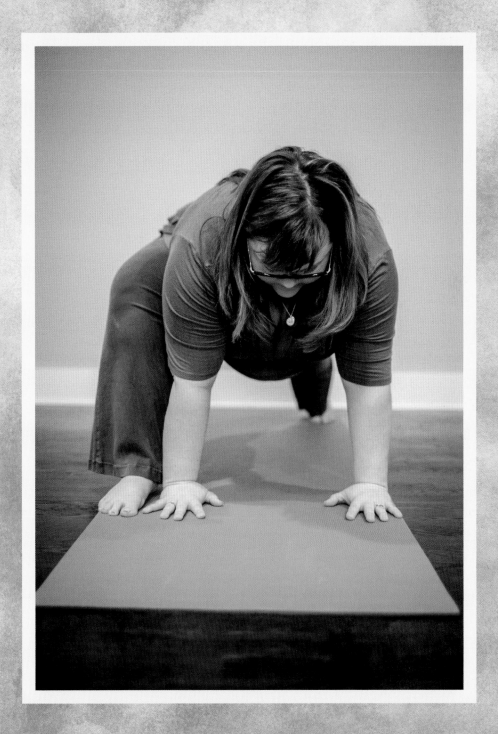

Child's Pose | *Balasana*

This pose is commonly offered as a resting option in yoga classes. But as traditionally taught, it is uncomfortable for many curvy bodies, often due to a lack of space for the belly. Though, there are ways to make it more comfortable.

Begin in Tabletop (on hands and knees) with your knees wide. Feel free to place a blanket under your knees as a cushion.

Bring your big toes toward each other (even to touch) behind you so that your legs are making a "V" with the point of the "V" being at your big toes (but if the toes don't touch, that's fine).

From there, begin to sit your butt back toward your heels (you may not sit completely on your heels, but that's the direction you're going) while walking your hands forward. Arms are straight (with a microbend in the elbows to prevent them from locking) with palms pressing firmly into the ground (particularly underneath the root of the first finger and thumb), head releasing down. If the forehead does not come to the ground in line with the spine (i.e., not dropping the head down, with the crown of the head to the floor), widen the hands to make more space and/or bring the floor to you by placing the head on a blanket or block.

Child's Pose is also sometimes taught with arms by the sides, palms facing up. I do not prefer this option for many curvy bodies, though, because even with taking the knees wide as above, the head still may not come down comfortably to the floor once you don't have the pressure of the hands on the floor, and the arms by the sides can sometimes cause the head to roll forward, straining the neck. I recommend only trying the arms-by-the-sides version if you're very comfortable in the arms-forward version and even then going slowly and watching carefully for neck strain.

Application to other poses: You can use the principle of making more space for your belly by widening your legs in any other seated pose where you run into belly discomfort. In addition, you can use support (blanket) under the head when lying down anytime the head does not come to the ground comfortably, whether in a prone or supine position.

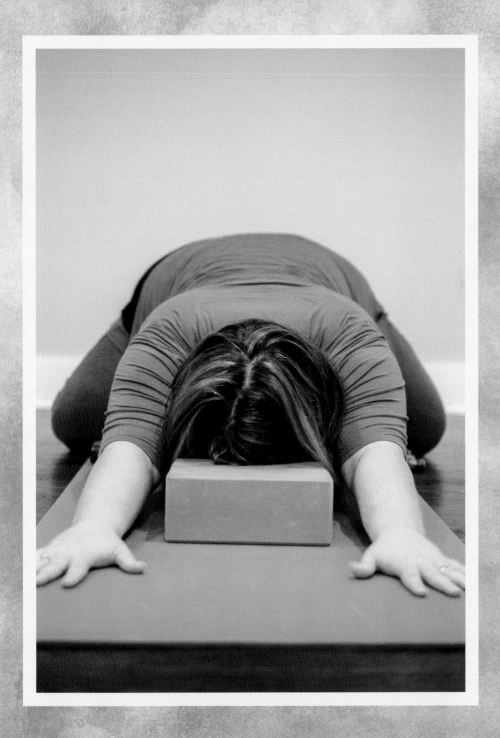

Warrior 1 | *Virabhadrasana I*

Begin standing in Mountain near the back of your mat with hands on hips.

Turn your left toes out about 30 degrees. *Another option*: Place this back heel against a baseboard or the bottom of the wall. This will give you some extra support in the pose and help you to work on alignment in the front leg as well as stability in the back leg.

And yet another option: Keep your left toes facing forward and come onto the ball of your foot. The beautiful thing about this option is that, because the hips are both facing forward, you alleviate any wonkiness if your hips are less open than you'd like them to be (and who isn't that true for?) or if they give you any problems.

Step your right foot forward a comfortable distance, approximately three feet.

Inhale and bend through your right knee, making sure your knee is aligned with your second toe. If you're bending past your ankle, move your front foot forward (or your back foot back) until you're not. As you do this, make sure that you are pressing firmly through the triangle of support under your back foot. The back foot has a tendency to roll in or out, which creates less stability and safety for the front leg, as well as the overall position.

Exhale and straighten your leg back to the starting position.

Repeat, moving on the breath two more times and using this as an opportunity to learn more about how far is good for your knee to bend today. After this, bend through the knee again and hold.

Once the legs are established in the pose, press your hands together in front of your heart if you feel stable. Another option is to lift your arms straight overhead, palms facing each other. Stay here for a couple breaths.

When you are ready to come out of the pose, bring your hands back to your hips. In one or more steps, step your back foot forward. Repeat on the other side.

Application to other poses: You can use the technique of more space between the feet (side-to-side) in other front-facing standing poses.

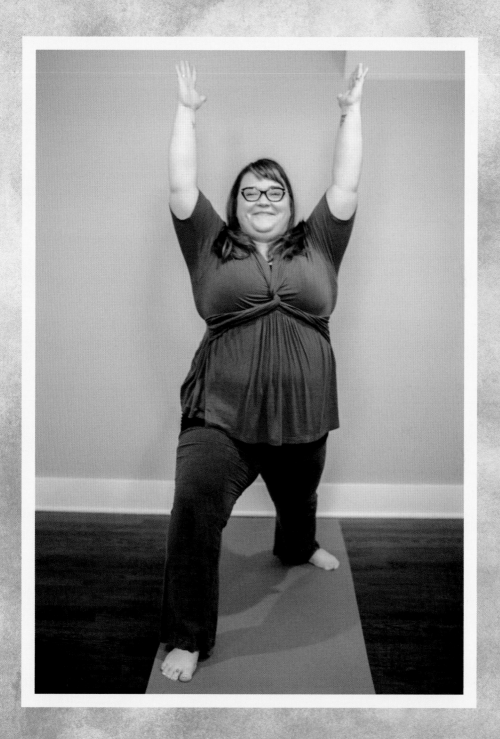

Side Angle | *Utthita Parsvakonasana*

Begin by standing on the mat with your feet a comfortabley wide distance apart, approximately three to four feet (1–1.2 m), hands on hips. If you're newer to yoga and/or have any foot/ankle issues, once you step your feet wide, step them in an inch or two (2–5 cm) for more stability if you've gone quite wide.

From here, turn your left toes in approximately 30 degrees and turn your right leg and foot out 90 degrees.

Bend through your right knee, making sure that your knee is pointing in the same direction as your second toe and that you're not bending past your ankle (if you are, move your front foot forward or your back foot back a bit until you're not). If your knee is not in line with your second toe, see if you can make it so. Sometimes that's not possible, though, often due to some kind of tightness in the hip or inner thigh. If the knee will not come into alignment, bend it less until it will. Keeping the knee aligned and safe is more important than bending more; favor alignment over depth in all of your poses, including this one.

Lengthen through your spine.

Bring your right hand to your right lower belly and move the belly a little to the middle, toward your belly button, as you keep your right side long. Next, bring your right forearm above your right knee. With your forearm above your knee, lift through your right side (so you don't collapse into your forearm/knee) as you roll your left shoulder up and back so that your chest faces the wall in front of you.

If you feel steady here, play with extending your left arm above and alongside your left ear, using the press of your back foot fully (especially through the pinky toe side) into the floor to reach more through the fingertips.

(continued)

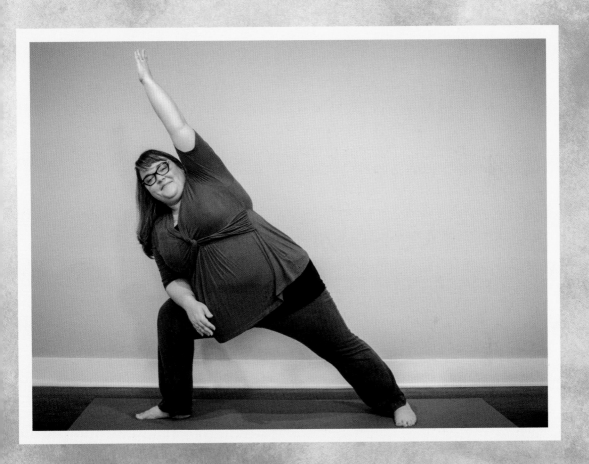

Side Angle | *Utthita Parsvakonasana*
(*continued*)

Your head stays in line with your spine, looking forward.

To come out of the pose, you might want to bring your right hand lightly above your right knee for support as you lift your torso up (if coming up directly doesn't work for you), then work your front leg toward straight. Either way, once you're up, turn both feet to parallel before repeating on the other side. If the feet feel tired, you might want to step them together for a moment before stepping them wide again and repeating on the other side.

Application to other poses: You can use the technique of moving the belly a little to the middle in any other poses where the belly may feel compressed at the side, such as twists (whether seated, standing, or lying down) or side bends.

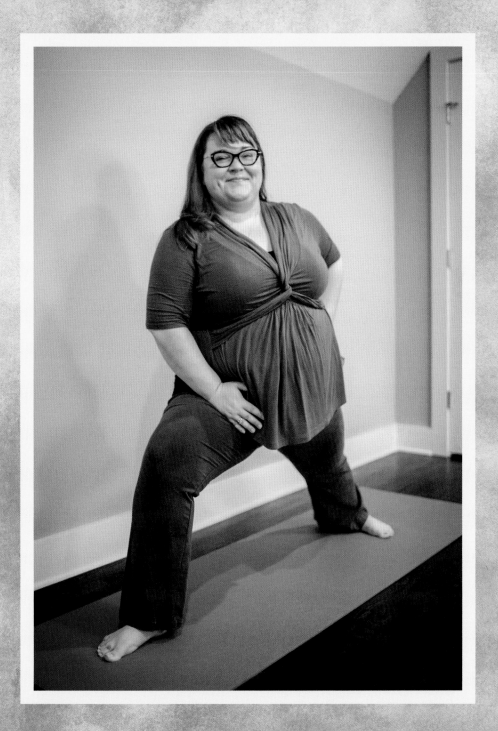

Triangle | *Trikonasana*

Begin by standing facing the long side of your mat with your hands on your hips. Place a block behind your right foot on the highest height.

Step your feet a comfortable wide distance apart, as in Side Angle. Bring your hands to your hips and turn your left toes in about 30 degrees. Turn your right leg and foot out 90 degrees.

Lengthen your spine and maintain that length as you bend your right knee and bring your right hand to a block behind your foot.

Begin working your right leg toward straight (emphasis on "toward"; just make it your version of straight for today).

Your left shoulder is likely still facing toward the ground here. So once you straighten your right leg, roll your left shoulder up and back, turning your torso to face the wall in front of you.

If and only if you feel stable here, play with lifting the left arm overhead, fingers pointing toward the ceiling. Make sure that both feet are pressing fully into the ground.

When you are ready to come out of the pose, bring the left hand back to the left hip if it's not there already. Bend slightly through the right knee and slowly come up to standing. Turn your feet back to parallel and repeat on the other side.

Application to other poses: You can use a block under the hand in any pose where the hand does not comfortably reach the floor. In addition, you can come into any straight-legged pose with a bent knee first and then work the leg toward straight.

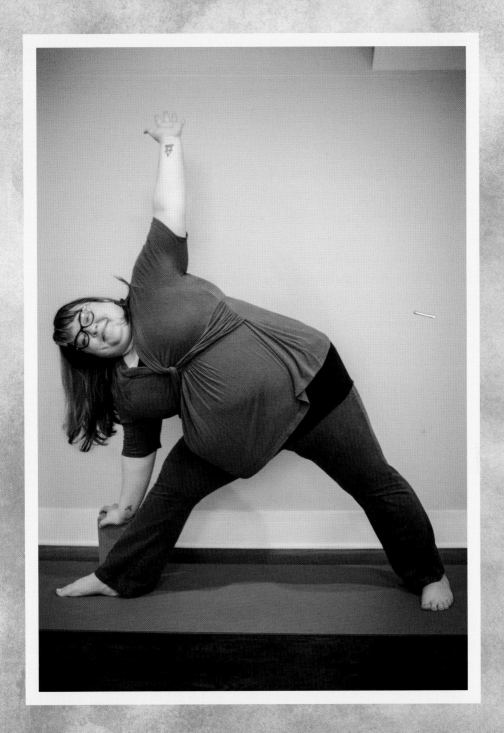

Tree | *Vrksasana*

Begin with the short end of your mat up against the wall.

Stand in front of the wall in Mountain Pose, with your back lightly against the wall (not mashing back, just in gentle contact), hands on hips.

From here, begin to shift your weight into your right leg. Be sure to have a microbend in this knee.

Next, bring your left heel above your inside right ankle bone; your left toes will be on the ground with your knee opening out toward the left, kind of like a kickstand. Consider how it feels to challenge your balance here with the support of the toes on the floor. If you're steady here, try this: press your hands together in front of your heart. And if that's steady for you, another option is to reach your arms overhead, palms facing each other.

Yet another option, either now or another time, is to lift the left foot off the floor and press it gently into your right calf (not your knee), left knee opening out. If you try this, press your foot into your calf as you press your calf into your foot. And another option over time, as you become comfortable with balancing at the wall, is to move yourself off the wall. I like to do this by starting with just moving an inch (2.5 cm) away. You're still off the wall even an inch (2.5 cm) away! But your mind is more comfortable because it knows it doesn't have far to go if you lose your balance.

In any of these options, you can also try bringing your hands in front of your chest, palms pressing together, or raising your arms overhead, palms facing each other.

To come out of this pose, bring your hands to your hips. Gently bring your left foot back to its starting position. Make any movements that would feel good to transition to the other side and repeat this pose there.

Application to other poses: You can use the wall for support in other balancing poses.

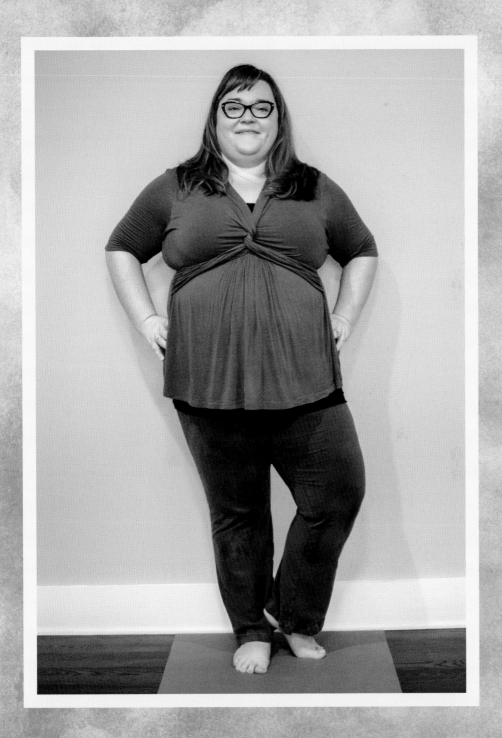

Simple Twist

Begin in Easy Seat, sitting up on a blanket. If that position doesn't work for you, you can also sit with your legs extended in front of you, taking the feet hip distance apart or a bit wider, as in Mountain Pose when standing.

Inhale and reach your arms overhead, palms facing each other. Exhale and move your hands into the position specified below:

Bring your left hand anywhere along your right leg it will reach, perhaps to your right knee. Bring your right hand to one of several places: (1) your right hip, (2) a block behind your right hip on any of the three heights, or (3) hand/fingertips on the ground. You want your hand to be somewhere that will help you maintain an extended spine and will keep your shoulders roughly in line with each other (in other words, one isn't slumping down while the other is arching up).

If your belly feels compressed, bring your right hand to your right lower belly and do one or more of the following: (1) move the belly down toward the hip crease; (2) move the belly up out of the hip crease; and/or (3) move the belly a little to the middle.

Using your breath, inhale and extend through your spine; exhale and twist any amount more, if possible. If your left arm feels stuck on your chest, lift it up and over, landing on the top part of the chest. You can also move the skin of the arm down and out, where it's in contact with the chest, to create some space. Additionally, you may find some parts of the belly are still a bit compressed now that you're in position, so feel free to use your left hand to move the belly a little to the middle once again.

After a few breaths when you're ready to switch sides, slowly unwind and come back to center. Repeat on the other side.

Application to other poses: You can use a block under the hand in any seated pose where the hands do not comfortably reach the floor, including Seated Forward Bends.

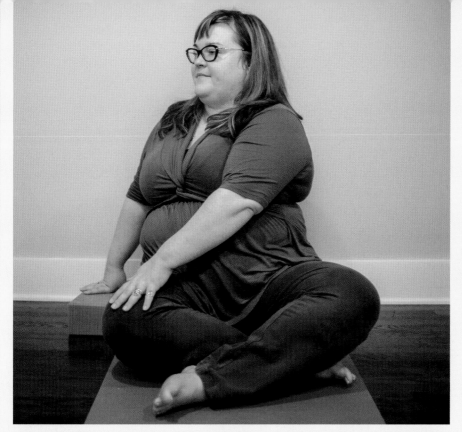

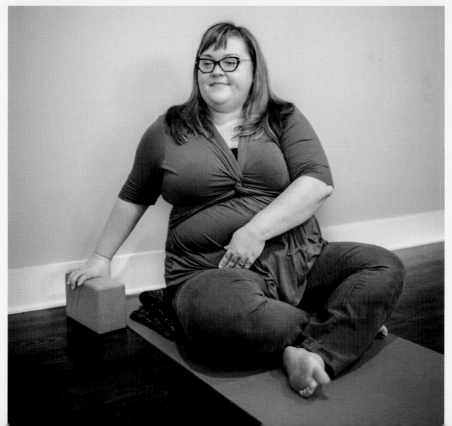

Marichi's Pose | *Marichyasana III*

Begin seated on a blanket with your legs extended in front of you and a block outside your right hip on the medium height. Take your right hand under your right hip and move the skin out and back, as in Easy Seat. Repeat on the other side.

Bend your right knee and draw it in toward your chest, bringing your foot to the floor. If you observe that your knee is bending out (that is, it isn't directly in line above your ankle), step your right foot a bit to the right until you can bring the knee into alignment.

Now bring your right hand to the right lower belly and move the skin a little to the middle so that it is less compressed between the torso and the thigh. Then lengthen your spine.

Reach your left arm up on an inhale. Exhale and wrap your left hand around your right knee, then bring your right hand to the block. Pause here and observe the relationship of your shoulders to each other. If the right shoulder is higher than the left, or you naturally have bend in your right elbow, you may be able to dial the block down or get rid of it, bringing your right fingertips or hand to the floor, depending on the length of your arms.

Inhale and lengthen your spine again; exhale and perhaps twist another little smidge, only ever taking advantage of available space, never forcing. Stay here for one to three breaths, then unwind yourself and repeat on the other side.

Application to other poses: You can use the hand holding onto the body anytime a body wrap of some kind (such as an elbow hooked outside a knee) would otherwise be used.

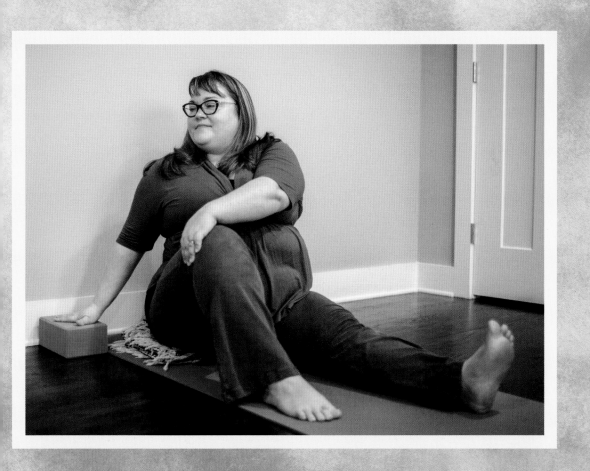

Seated Forward Bend |
Paschimottanasana

Begin seated on a blanket with your legs extending straight in front of you and one block on either side of your thighs on the medium height. Bring your right hand under your right hip and move the skin out and back, as in Easy Seat. Repeat on the other side. You may also want to move the skin of the inner thighs as in Easy Seat.

Just for a moment here, inhale and reach your arms overhead. Exhale and fold forward over your legs, observing how far forward you comfortably can go and if/where your belly feels compressed. Then come out of the forward bend, back to seated.

Now we'll try a two-part experiment.

Part One: Bring your hands to either side of your lower belly. Press the belly in toward your torso as you move it down toward or into your hip crease (similar to the action we already discussed in Standing Forward Bend). Keeping your hands here, inhale and lengthen your spine; exhale, fold forward again. Once you move as far forward as available with an extended spine, you can then release your hands to the blocks on any height. You will likely need to move them down from your hips. If the blocks are on the low height and you naturally have bend in your elbows, you may be able to remove the blocks and bring your hands to the floor. Notice the following: How does this version of the pose feel in comparison to the first time you did the pose? How far forward are you able to come, and how does your belly feel? Make a mental note, then come back out.

Part Two: Again bring your hands to either side of your lower belly. This time, though, take a gentle hold of the belly and lift it up out of the hip crease. As you continue to hold, inhale and lengthen your spine; exhale and fold forward. Once you've come forward, you can release your hands to wherever they naturally fall, placing them on blocks on any height if they don't reach the floor comfortably. Once again, ask yourself:

(continued)

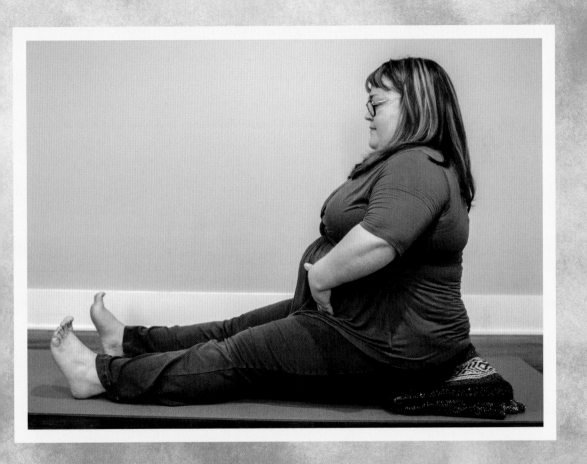

Seated Forward Bend |
Paschimottanasana (continued)

How does this version of the pose compare to the first version? And the second? If one of the belly moves helped you come in further and/or more comfortably, make a mental note of it so you can use it any time you do a Seated Forward Bend.

Application to other poses: You can move the belly down, up, or to the middle in any pose, seated, standing, or lying down, where the belly feels compressed and moving it would make you feel more comfortable and/or enable you to come further into the pose.

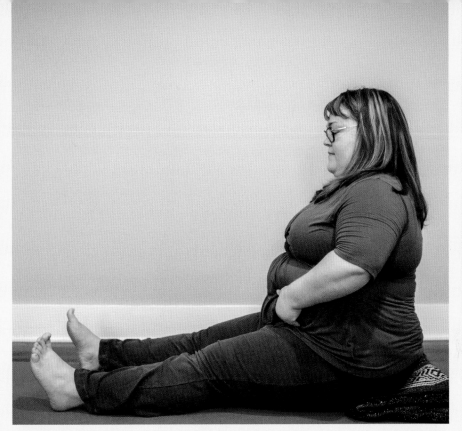

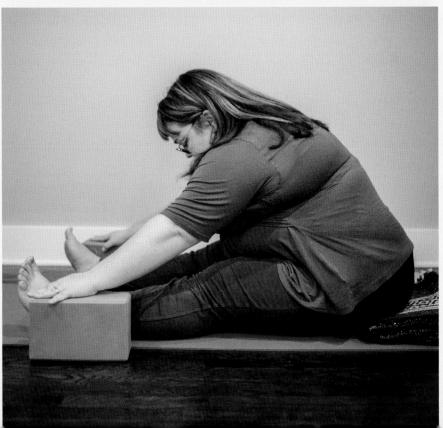

Pigeon | *Kapotasana*

Pigeon on the Floor with Support

Begin seated with your legs in front of you. Have a blanket nearby and two blocks in front of you.

Bring your right shin roughly parallel to the front edge of your mat. Let your right foot be a bit closer to your pelvis than the front left corner of the mat. Take your right thumb into the crook behind your right knee and use it to roll the skin out toward the shin. This allows the knee to close a bit more and can make the flesh of the calf feel less compressed.

Next, take your right hand outside your right hip and begin to shift yourself into your right hip, letting the left leg get ready to move. Then, briefly tuck your left lower leg beside your left hip, in what is sometimes known as a "Z-sit." This is a great seated version of Pigeon; feel free to stay here (walking the hands forward as below if desired). Now, bring your torso back to center as you bring both your hands in front of your right shin to blocks or the floor. Once your hands are steady, come onto your left knee briefly, getting it ready to move behind you (if this is not comfortable, keep the left leg extended as it was and stay here).

If you'd like, another option is to begin to move your left leg directly back behind you, ending up with the entire front of the lower leg and much of the front of the upper leg in contact with the floor.

From here, tuck your folded blanket underneath your right hip so it is supported (if it's not already in contact with the floor). If the blanket isn't folded tall enough, fold it so that it is or add another blanket.

Hands can stay where they are, though you may want to briefly use one of your hands to move your belly to the middle, particularly on your right side. You may also want to fold forward further, either walking the blocks further away from you or resting onto them here.

When you are ready to come out of the pose, shift your weight slightly to your right until you can get your left leg free enough to move it to the left enough to come around to seated. Give yourself a moment here, then repeat on the other side.

(continued)

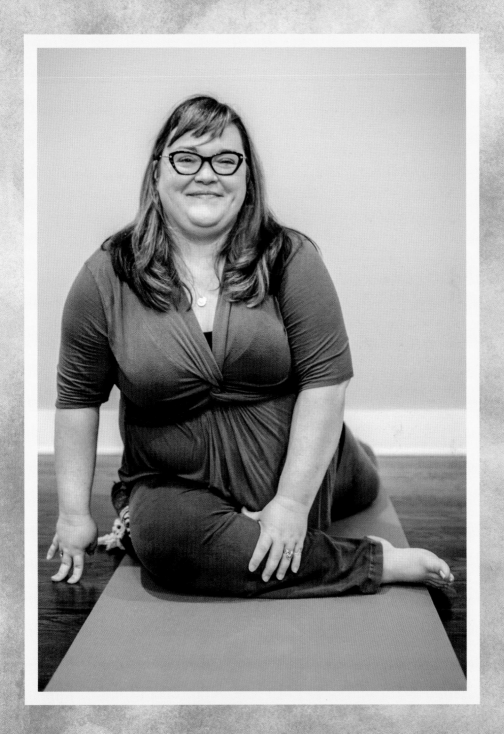

Pigeon | *Kapotasana* (continued)

Pigeon with Bolster and Chair

Place a stable chair at the top of your mat, with the seat facing you. Place a bolster two to three feet (61–91 cm) in front of the chair, parallel to the top (short) edge of your mat.

There are two ways to come in. (1) Come to hands and knees on the mat, behind the bolster. Step your right foot forward, in front of the bolster. Then, move your right foot to the left, allowing your right lower leg to come down. From here, bring your hands to the chair seat to help as you begin to move your left leg back behind you, extending it as far as is comfortable, ending up with the back of the right hip and the front of the left hip in contact with the bolster.

(2) Sit on the bolster, with your legs in the space between the bolster and the chair. Place your hands on the chair seat as you begin to move your right leg to be parallel to the short edge of the mat, as in step 1. Keeping the hands on the chair seat, begin to shift into your right hip so that your left leg has room to move. Bring your left lower leg beside you in a Z-sit, as in the previous version of Pigeon, then move it back behind you. Finally, move the torso back to center.

No matter if you came into position through step 1 or step 2, pause here with your hands on the chair seat. Inhale and lengthen your spine; exhale and fold forward any amount, perhaps folding your arms on the chair seat and resting your head down. You can move the chair closer to you if you want more support; the opposite is also true.

When you are ready to come out of the pose, bring your hands to the chair seat. Shift into your right hip to free up your left leg enough to move it to the left until you can come around to a seated position. Then repeat on the other side.

Application to other poses: You can use a blanket and/or a bolster under one or both hips in any pose where they do not comfortably reach the floor. In addition, you can roll the skin of the calf in any pose where there is thigh/calf compression.

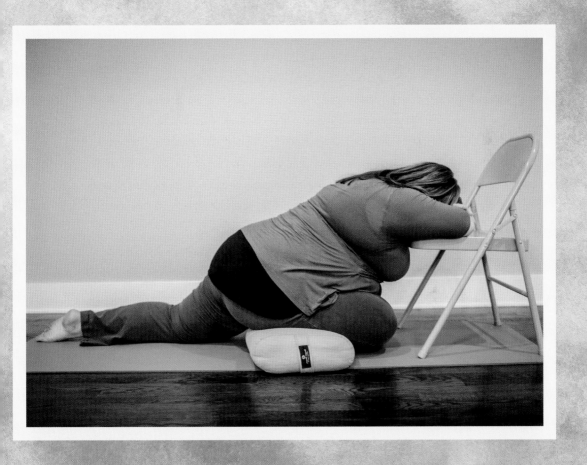

Knees to Chest | *Apanasana*

Lie on your back and begin with your knees bent and your feet flat on the floor.

Keeping your head in contact with the ground (not straining the neck by lifting it up), slowly draw your right knee in toward your chest. Hands can be anywhere here: on top of the knee, around the knee, or behind the thigh.

If the hands do not comfortably reach the legs, grab a strap and loop it around the ball of one foot (you can also do this before you lie down if you know you'll want it ahead of time). With the strap on the foot, extend that leg and lift it from the floor—anywhere from 30 to 90 degrees. Once the leg is extended, bring your other foot to meet the foot inside the strap so that both feet are in the strap, next to each other. Lift both legs as close to 90 degrees as is comfortable, then gently slip the strap off the feet, behind your legs, pulling the strap toward your legs as you do. You want the strap to catch just below the knee. Once it does, bend both knees, walk your hands down the strap as needed so you can hold close to the knees, and hug your knees in to your chest.

Whether using the strap or not, hug the knees in a comfortable amount. Sometimes taking the knees a bit wider can give space to the belly if it feels too compressed, but there is some belly compression naturally in this pose.

When you are ready to come out of the pose, gently release the strap and/ or your hands and bring one foot to the ground, followed by the other.

Application to other poses: You can use a strap behind the knees in any other poses where one or both knees are hugged toward the chest.

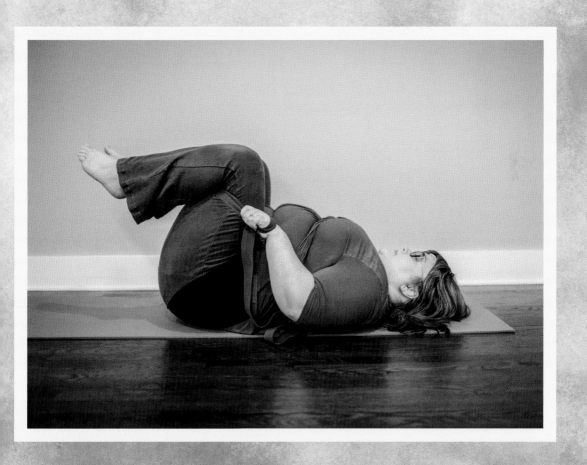

Bridge | *Setu Bandha Sarvangasana*

Bridge Pose has a gentle inversion quality to it. An inversion is a pose where the head is below the heart. For some people in inversions, the skin of the chest falls forward into the throat or face, which is uncomfortable at best and suffocating/strangling at worst. If you anticipate or experience this issue in inversions, try this:

While sitting down (or standing up, but before you lie down on your mat), bring a yoga strap behind your back so that you can hold an end in each hand.

Move the strap so that the back of it is approximately in line with your shoulder blades.

Buckle your strap (this process is different depending on what kind of strap you have) and cinch it in at the top of your chest. Remember, the goal is to keep the skin of the chest from falling into your face when you're upside down, so having the strap at the middle of your chest isn't helpful.

Check that the strap is secure and comfortable and that the buckle won't be digging into your skin. Now you are ready to practice your Bridge.

Lie on your back on your mat (no blanket under the head for this one). Bend your knees and press your feet into the floor.

Bring your feet so they are parallel with each other, approximately hip-distance apart.

Walk your feet in toward your butt a smidge—probably an inch (2.5 cm) or so.

Inhale and begin to lift your hips off the ground any amount. Exhale and slowly lower them back down. Continue this movement for five more breaths, perhaps coming up a little higher each time.

On your next inhale, lift your hips up and hold the pose here for two breaths.

Once you are done, lower back down slowly.

Application to other poses: You can use the strap around the chest in any other inversions where suffocation/strangulation may be felt.

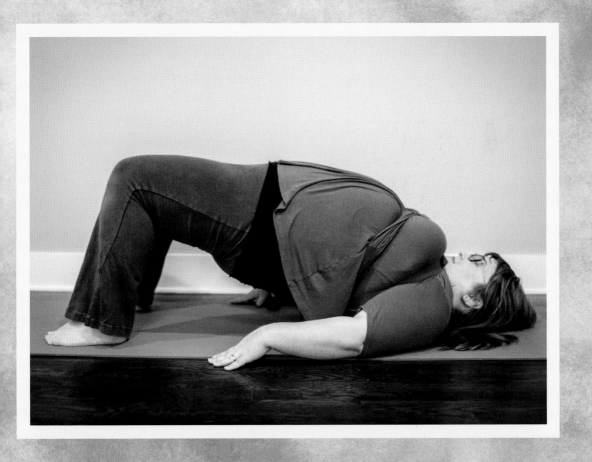

Cobra | *Bhujangasana*

You might like to start with a blanket nearby.

Baby Cobra

Begin by lying on your belly. Before you do anything else, tuck your toes under and walk your legs back however far they'll go (usually about an inch [2.5 cm]). This makes space for the skin of the thighs/belly to rest more comfortably, thus also allowing the low back to be more comfortable and aligned. If your chest feels compressed, bring your hands to either side and move the skin out to its respective side to make a little space and feel less direct compression.

Bring your hands under your shoulders and hug your elbows in toward your torso. On an inhale, lightly draw your navel toward your spine and begin to lift up from your sternum, keeping your head in line with your spine. This brings you into a gentle backbend using the core and back to come up, not so much the hands. The hands are so lightly pressing into the floor here that you could almost lift them up for a second.

When you come down, rest your forehead down to release the neck. You can rest it on the floor if it comes down comfortably, but, if not, rest it on your crossed arms, stacked fists, or a blanket.

Cobra

Cobra starts off the same way as Baby Cobra, so repeat the beginning steps to come into position.

The difference comes once you get an inch or two (2–5 cm) off the ground. From here, press a bit more firmly through the hands and reach forward and up more through the chest. The glutes can be engaged here but not extremely tightly clinched.

When you are done, lower down slowly and rest the forehead down.

Application to other poses: You can tuck the legs under and walk them back before doing any prone yoga pose.

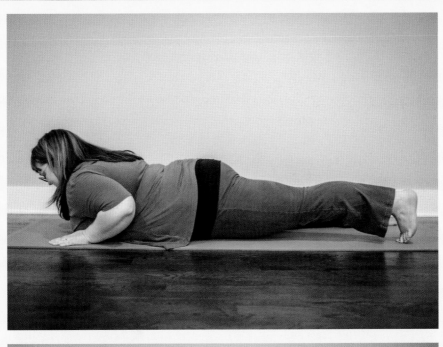

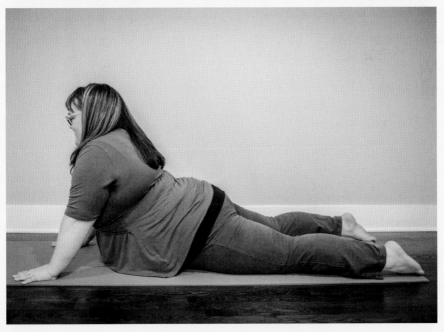

Reclining Hand-to-Big-Toe | *Supta Padangusthasana*

Begin seated on your mat, legs extended in front of you.

Loop your strap around the ball of your right foot, then bring both sides of the strap into your right hand. Keeping the strap around your foot, gently come to a position lying down on your back, knees bent with feet flat on the floor.

Have one side of the strap in each hand. Inhale and lift your right foot and leg overhead with the strap, keeping your knee bent. Exhale and pause here. Begin to work your leg toward straight.

The left knee can be bent here. Alternatively, the left leg could be extended on the ground. If your left leg is extended on the ground, make sure that it stays there. Sometimes it wants to pop up and be sort of bent and sort of straight, which can jeopardize your knee and lower back.

There are several ways to hold the strap. You can grip it with fists or you can wrap it around your hand as shown in the photo. Additionally, you can hold it closer to your torso with elbows bent or closer to your foot with arms extended.

When you are ready to switch sides, bring your left foot to meet your right inside the strap, either directly up in the air or you can bring the right leg down first (even to the floor). This is usually the simplest way to switch feet. When the left foot is secure, slowly release the right foot from the strap and lower it back to the ground.

Repeat on the other side. When you are ready to come out of the pose completely, release the strap from the foot and lower the leg back to the ground.

Application to other poses: You can use the technique of getting the strap on your foot before lying down in any reclined pose with a strap. In addition, you can use the strap in any pose where your arms would benefit from an extension.

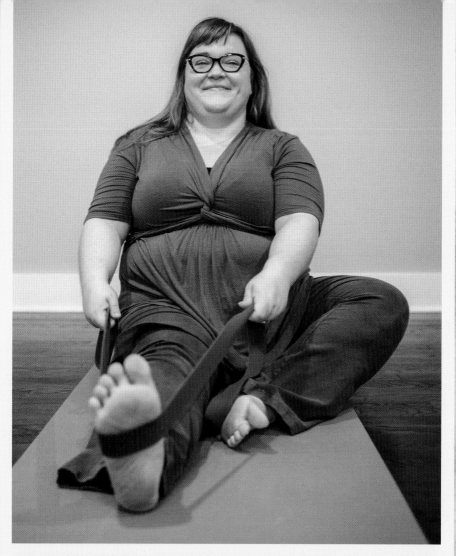

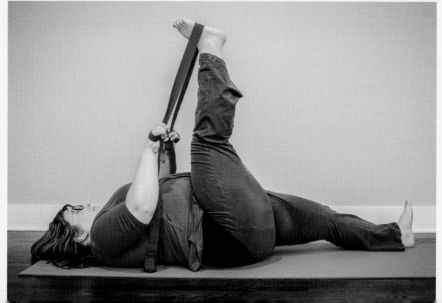

Legs Up the Wall | *Viparita Karani*

To begin, come to a seated position with your right side perpendicular to the wall. You want your right hip as close to the wall as possible, even on the wall. Once you come into the pose, it's much easier to scoot away if you're too close than it is to scoot in if you're too far away.

Place your left hand on the mat outside your hip and walk it away from you. As you do, allow your torso to lie down with it so that you end up with your upper body on its side.

Next, begin to roll onto your back, allowing your legs to slide up the wall as you do. If you feel a bit awkward, you're not alone! It *is* awkward, especially the first few times you do it. But once you get in, it can be nice!

Once you are here, observe how your hamstrings (the backs of the thighs) feel. If they feel overstretched, bend your knees, place your feet on the wall, and scoot yourself half an inch (13 mm) away, then reassess. If you find you need to be more than an inch or two (2-5 cm) away, the option below with the chair may be best for now so you don't risk hyperextending your knees.

To do this pose on a chair, sit in front of a chair (chair seat facing you with its back to a wall). You come into the pose the exact same way; the only difference is your lower legs rest on the chair seat rather than your entire leg on the wall.

No matter what version of the pose you're in, your arms can rest wherever is comfortable. If it feels as if your forehead is tipping backwards, even a little bit, try the chin tuck as described in *Savasana* below and/or place a blanket under your head.

When you are ready to come out of the pose, bend your knees and press your feet into the wall. Pause here and then roll slowly to one side (yes, it's just as graceful coming out as it was going in!). Then gently bring yourself up to a seated position.

Application to other poses: You can use a chair to modify just about any pose.

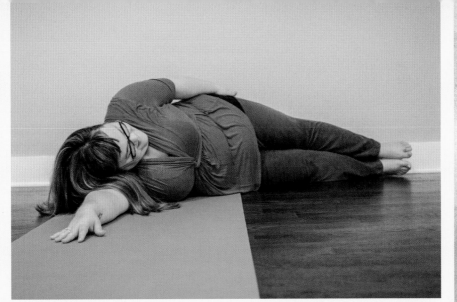

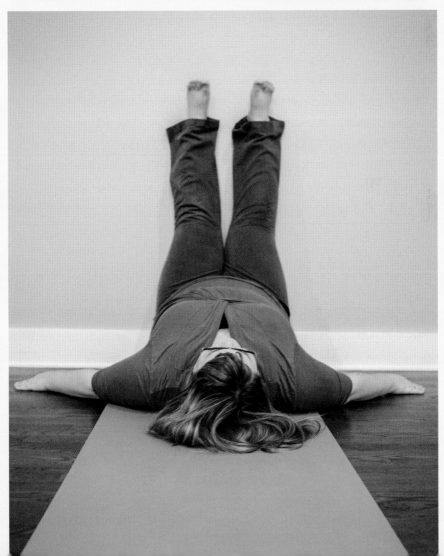

Final Relaxation (Corpse) | *Savasana*

Place a folded blanket at the top of your mat. Lie down on your back with your head on the blanket, knees bent, and your feet on the floor.

If you know you have lower back discomfort when you lie on the floor, try these options. (1) Step your feet an inch (2–5 cm) or so closer toward your hips and press your feet down firmly. On an inhale, lift your hips up and bring your hands to the back of your hips. Breathe at your own pace here as you gently tuck your tailbone while using your hands to move the flesh of the hips down toward your feet. Once you do that, slowly lower your hips back down. This creates a little more space for the lower back. (2) To get more space to the lower back coming from the upper part of the spine now, gently lift your head an inch (2–5 cm) or so off the ground so you can bring your hands to the back of your head. Tuck your chin lightly toward your chest, just using your hands to support your head, not to force your chin down. Keep the chin tucked as you lower your head back down and remove your hands.

From here, you can begin to slowly extend your legs and see how you feel. If your lower back is still uncomfortable, try placing a bolster or a rolled-up blanket underneath your knees. This is yet another way to create more space for the lower back.

If you are still not comfortable, make your way into any position that is comfortable for you. The purpose of this pose is to ease you into a state of light conscious awareness and relaxation, so you want to be comfortable!

Once you are in a position that works for you, take five deep breaths, taking your time. Next, turn your attention to your feet and begin a body check-in, as in Chapter Two of this book. When you complete the body check-in, expand your awareness through your whole body and let yourself rest here for as long as you'd like. So that your mind doesn't have to worry about the time, you might like to set a timer for the length of time you'd like to stay here (just make sure it doesn't have a blaring alarm!).

(continued)

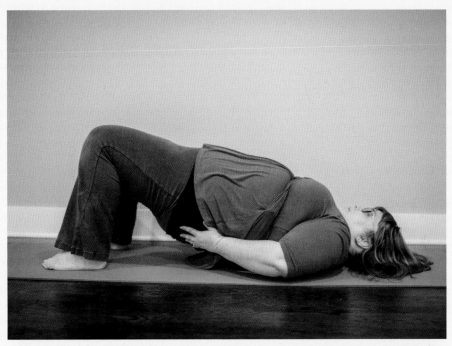

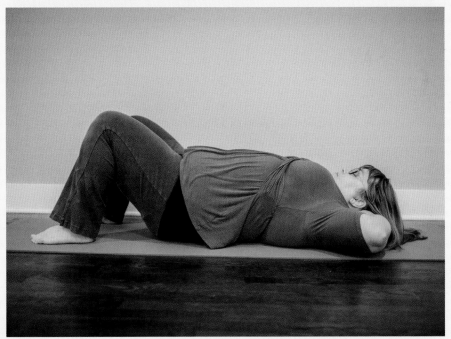

Final Relaxation (Corpse) | *Savasana*
(*continued*)

Whenever you decide to come out of the pose, take a moment to notice how you feel. You might even like to name that feeling to yourself in a word or a short phrase. Noticing and naming how you feel is one way to deepen your understanding of your bodily experience from moment to moment. This is also a wonderful time to do the practice—presence, get curious, challenge, and affirm.

You can then begin to invite some movement back into your body by wiggling your fingers and toes. Make any movements that would feel good, perhaps reaching arms overhead and getting a long stretch through the whole body.

When you're ready, roll slowly to one side and rest there for a few breaths, perhaps using your bottom arm as a pillow. As it feels good, roll over a bit more until you can bring your top hand to the floor, then slowly press yourself up to a seated position, bringing your head up last.

Application to other poses: You can create space in the back in any supine pose by lifting the hips/moving the skin and lifting the head/tucking the chin. In addition, support under the knees and/or head may be useful in other supine poses (except for Bridge, where the head needs more space).

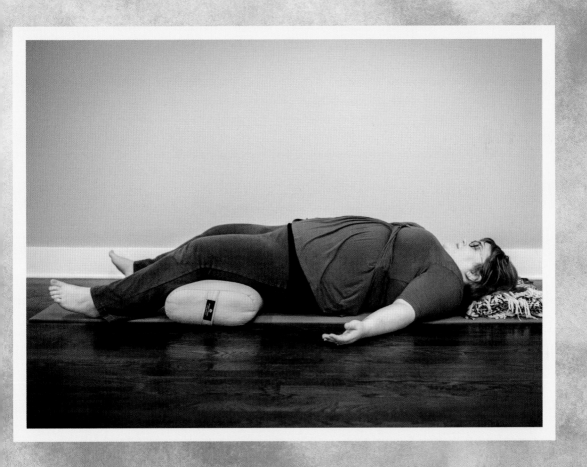

Acknowledgments

When people ask me how Curvy Yoga came into being, I always say it wouldn't exist without our community of kind, loving, brilliant folks who are committed to the continual discovery process of what it means to get to know, like, and maybe even love their bodies through yoga. I'm inspired by the ways y'all show up for yourselves—and each other!—every day. Also, I couldn't be more humbled by the myriad ways you support and encourage me. This book is my love letter to and for each of you.

Special thanks go to all the yoga teachers who have added Curvy Yoga to their teaching repertoire. I deeply believe in sharing Curvy Yoga through local teachers and communities, and I couldn't be happier that teachers have taken up the banner of body-affirming yoga all over the world. My hat is forever off to you and all you do to open the doors of yoga to people of every shape and size.

And to the members of our virtual studio as well as my local students in Nashville, wow. I like to think of my heart as having lots of pockets where I tuck people and memories that are important to me. Y'all occupy a very large pocket indeed!

It turns out that what they say is true: Writing a book is hard! And it takes at least as much emotional labor as anything else. I am so grateful for my patient and kind agent, Monika Verma, who has had my back every step of the way. Thank you also to my editor Kate Zimmermann and the great team at Sterling for bringing this book to life. Working with smart women is the best! Thanks and love to Diana Ventimiglia for believing in this book. Thanks also go to Alexandra Franzen for her help with the very earliest ideas for this book, as well as Laurie Wagner for her kind eyes reading an early draft and reassuring me that I didn't have to delete the whole thing and start over and Stephanie Hagen for her help with ideas for the cover.

Big love goes to my dear friends Pleasance Silicki and Jennifer Louden for supporting me through the process of writing this book, often on a near-daily basis.

When I didn't believe I could do it, they did, and that gave me enough energy to keep going. I wish for everyone friends like this!

Without Melissa Montilla and Tzahi Moskovitz somehow believing I had what it took to be part of their yoga teacher-training program years ago, this book would not exist. Though I had no clue what I was doing at the time, and was too scared to talk about my dream of teaching a class like the yet-to-be-named Curvy Yoga, they supported me, and I will always be grateful to have landed in such a loving space with them and my wonderful fellow students. Marianne Elliott believed in the work I was doing from the very early days and helped me do the same.

Speaking of fellow students, the friends I have made through my yoga practice have been some of my most influential teachers. The way I see them embodying their yoga on and off the mat inspires me endlessly. Much love to Barbara Denowh, Nancy Alder, Melanie Klein, and Jane House in this regard—and all others. And my online colleagues, who are also my real-life friends, keep me grounded, connected, and laughing—such important parts of life! Much gratitude to Rachel Cole, Mara Glatzel, Racheal Cook, Vivienne McMaster, and Margarita Tartakovsky. I'm also grateful for my fellow teachers in this body-affirming realm, particularly those who came before me: Abby Lentz, Michael Hayes, Meera Patricia Kerr, Sally Pugh, Lanita Varshell, and Megan Stancill.

The real magic behind the scenes of Curvy Yoga comes from our team: Erin Blaskie, Crystal McLeod, and Liz Eskridge. These genius women have my back when things are good as well as when things are overwhelming (and they somehow still want to work with me) and they are each true friends. Most importantly, though, they make sure all our students are well cared for. I'm so blessed to have worked with them for years, and I hope to continue to into the future! Thank you also to Emily and Brandon Gnetz, a dream team who keep our photos and videos on point (Emily took the photos for this book!).

I wouldn't have had the courage to create Curvy Yoga at all, or do much of anything really, without two of the loves of my life: my sister, Julia Zeal, and my best friend, Nora Spencer-Loveall. When I can't see who I am anymore, they remind me. I also want to thank my mom for growing with me in this realm of body acceptance and being proud of the work I do.

For a long time I never thought I'd find love, at least not until those Overnight Weight Loss pills kicked in and I woke up with a new body. So what a gift when I met Nic Guest-Jelley and he loved me for me. You really can't ask for more than that, can you? Except maybe a partner who's also a great editor and can help make your book at least 1,000 percent better—oh but wait, he's that, too! I'd sail away with him any day.

DON'T FORGET
to share
YOUR
compassion
WITH
yourself

Resources

To learn more about Curvy Yoga, visit www.CurvyYoga.com.

To receive and download audio versions of the practices in this book, as well as videos of the poses in action, visit www.curvyyoga.com/book.

Notes

Preface

1. http://www.theatlantic.com/health/archive/2016/06/you-cant-willpower-your-way-to-lasting-weight-loss/488801/.

Chapter One: Twenty Years. Sixty-five Diets. No Results. Or How We Got Here

1. http://fortune.com/2015/05/22/lean-times-for-the-diet-industry/.

2. http://brenebrown.com/.

3. http://nymag.com/scienceofus/2015/10/why-weight-watchers-doesnt-work.html?mid=fb-share-scienceofus.

4. http://www.healthyhorns.utexas.edu/n_bodyimage.html.

5. https://www.washingtonpost.com/news/wonk/wp/2015/05/04/why-diets-dont-actually-work-according-to-a-researcher-who-has-studied-them-for-decades/.

Chapter Three: Get Curious: Finding the Voices in Your Head That You Can Trust

1. Evelyn Tribole and Elyse Resch, *Intuitive Eating: A Revolutionary Program That Works*, 3rd ed. (New York: St. Martin's Griffin, 2012).

2. https://www.intuitiveeating.com/content/what-intuitive-eating.

Chapter Four: Challenge What You Know. (Yes, I Mean Everything.)

1. http://www.theguardian.com/lifeandstyle/2014/dec/05/detox-myth-health-diet-science-ignorance.

2. http://haescommunity.com/.

3. Linda Bacon, *Health at Every Size: The Surprising Truth about Your Weight* (Dallas: BenBella Books, 2010, 5).

4. http://www.nytimes.com/2016/05/08/opinion/sunday/why-you-cant-lose-weight-on-a-diet.html?_r=0.
   5. http://www.nytimes.com/2015/11/29/opinion/sunday/could-your-healthy-diet-make-me-fat.html.

6. http://www.prevention.com/health/healthy-living/weight-and-obesity-discrimination-doctors.

7. Mark Singleton, *Yoga Body: The Origins of Modern Posture Practice* (New York: Oxford University Press, 2010).

8. Melanie Klein and Anna Guest-Jelley, *Yoga and Body Image: 25 Personal Stories About Beauty, Bravery & Loving Your Body* (Woodbury, MN: Llewellyn Publications, 2014).

9. http://self-compassion.org/about/.

10. https://www.intuitiveeating.com/content/warning-dieting-increases-your-risk-gaining-more-weight-update.

Chapter Five: Affirm/Trust Me, This Is Way More Practical Than It Sounds

1. Nicolai Bachman, *The Path of the Yoga Sutras: A Practical Guide to the Core of Yoga* (Louisville, CO: Sounds True, 2011, 1).

2. Donna Farhi, *Yoga Mind, Body & Spirit: A Return to Wholeness* (New York: Henry Holt, 2000).

3. Leslie Kaminoff and Amy Matthews, *Yoga Anatomy*, 2nd ed. (Champaign, IL: Human Kinetics, 2012).

4. Megan Garcia, *Mega Yoga: The First Yoga Program for Curvy Women* (New York: Dorling Kindersley, 2006).

Appendix: Yoga Poses Should Work for You, Not the Other Way Around

1. www.curvyyoga.com/location-select.

Index

(Continued on following page)